AF334537

A Practical Clinical Guide to Resin Cements

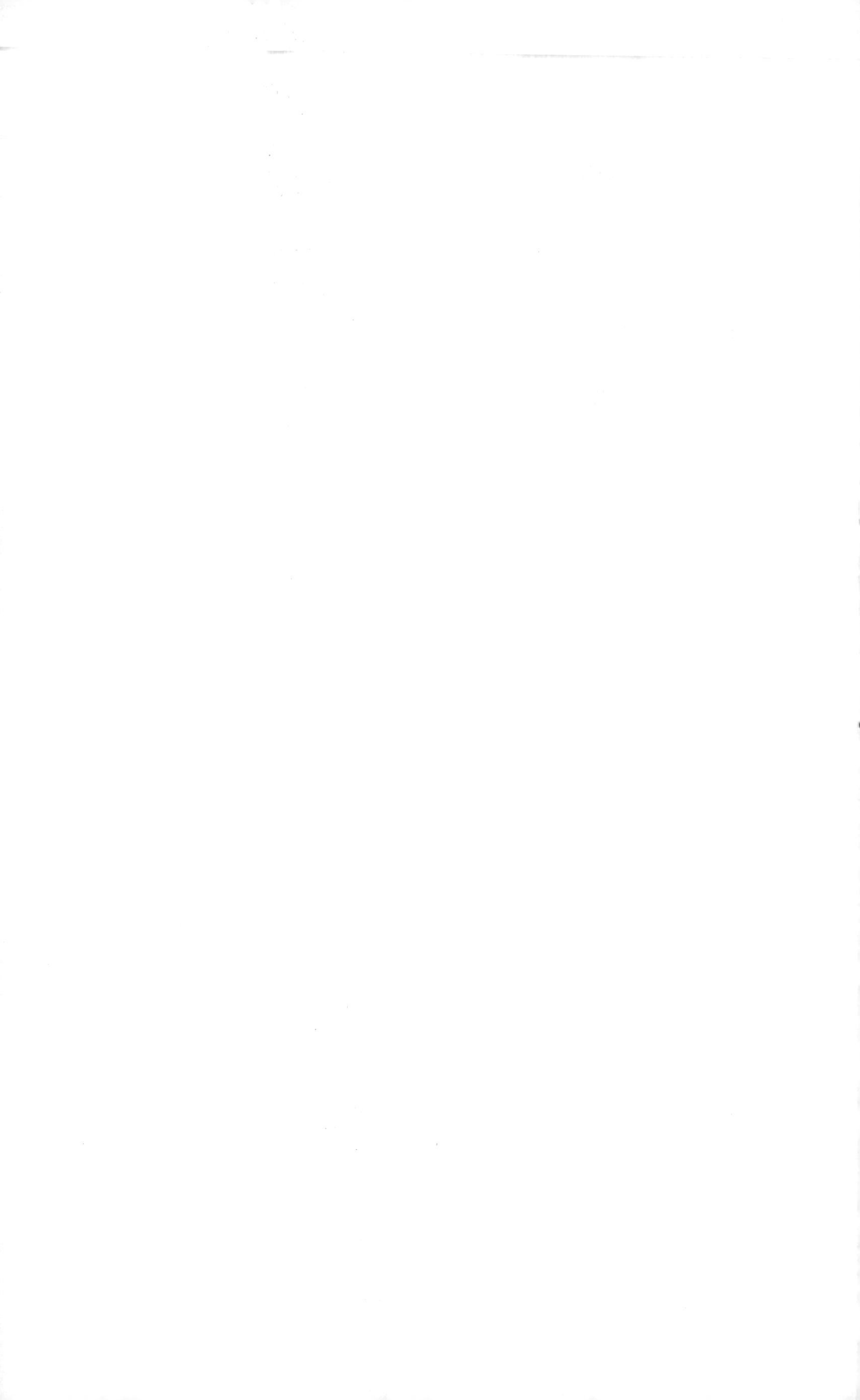

Michelle Sunico-Segarra • Armin Segarra

A Practical Clinical Guide to Resin Cements

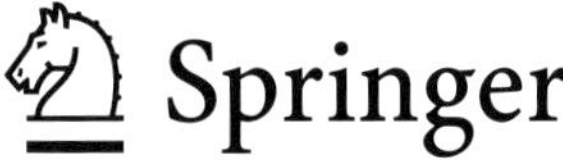

Michelle Sunico-Segarra
University of the Philippines
Manila College of Dentistry
Paranaque
Philippines

Armin Segarra
University of the Philippines
Manila College of Dentistry
Paranaque
Philippines

ISBN 978-3-662-43841-1   ISBN 978-3-662-43842-8   (eBook)
DOI 10.1007/978-3-662-43842-8
Springer Heidelberg New York Dordrecht London

Library of Congress Control Number: 2014951827

Printed on acid-free paper

Springer is part of Springer Science+Business Media (www.springer.com)

Preface

This book is a simplified guide to the cementation of indirect restorations with resin cements. With the many types and proprietary brands of resin cements in the market today, it is easy to get confused with which cement to use for a particular situation. The purpose of this book is to guide the clinician in choosing the right resin cement for a particular case and to give simple and clinical pointers in cementation.

Most of the information that is found in this book does not depict the authors' ideas, as this book is merely a compilation of knowledge learned from lectures from well-known authors and lecturers; from actual lectures, workshops, books, journal articles, articles from the Internet, dental forum, and group discussions; and from clinical pearls that have been learned along the way from the authors' years of dental practice.

This book is divided into two parts. The first part is an in-depth discussion of technical information about luting cements in general and resin cements in particular. This part is theoretical and academic and cites numerous studies regarding resin cements and serves as the foundation and theoretical background for the second part, which is the clinical part. The second part can stand alone and deals with clinical tips and procedural guidelines on cementation with resin cements. The reader may choose to skip the first part and proceed immediately to the second part of the book for an easy-to-understand, step-by-step clinical guide to cementation.

<table>
<tr><td>Paranaque, Philippines</td><td align="right">Michelle Sunico-Segarra</td></tr>
<tr><td>Paranaque, Philippines</td><td align="right">Armin Segarra</td></tr>
</table>

Contents

Part II   Clinical Aspects of Resin Cements

Part I

Theoretical and Technical Background

The Evolution of Cements for Indirect Restorations from Luting to Bonding

1

1.1 Introduction

In indirect restorations such as crowns, bridges, inlays, onlays, and posts, cement plays a vital link between the restoration and the tooth. Although the retention of crowns, bridges, inlays, and onlays depends primarily on friction between the walls of the preparation and the internal surface of the restoration, the cement is still an integral part of the indirect restoration assembly.

Different types of cement have been used over the past 100 years. The earliest cements did not have any adhesive properties. They merely filled the microscopic space between the walls of the preparation and the internal surface of the indirect restoration, hence the term luting cements or conventional cements. Luting cements include the zinc phosphate cements, polycarboxylates and the glass ionomers. They have performed particularly well on restorations with long, almost parallel walls as retention mainly relied on the frictional forces between the walls of the preparation and the internal wall of the restoration.

Over the years, indirect restorations have evolved. Newer materials have been developed to fabricate indirect restorations such as composite-ceramic hybrid materials (ceromers) and high-strength ceramics among others. Retention of indirect restorations became more complicated because of the increased complexity of these materials. These tooth-colored materials require cements that have better physical and mechanical properties. In addition, indirect restorations with compromised retention such as short crowns, tooth preparations with too much divergence, and too little remaining tooth structures are not retained well with conventional cements.

To keep up with these developments, newer cements were developed such as the resin hybrid cements and resin cements. The newest of these cements, the resin cements, have adhesive properties and have true adhesion to the internal surface of the restoration and to the tooth structure. These cements are not merely luting but bonding cements.

© Springer-Verlag Berlin Heidelberg 2015

M. Sunico-Segarra, A. Segarra, *A Practical Clinical Guide to Resin Cements*,

DOI 10.1007/978-3-662-43842-8_1

Today, cements used for indirect restorations are divided into two main types: the older luting cements which do not require any pretreatment and the newer bonding cements.

1.2   Luting Cements

1.2.1   Zinc Phosphate Cements

The oldest of the luting cements, zinc phosphate, has been used for over 100 years. Zinc phosphate is a mixture of zinc oxide powder and phosphoric acid liquid. The initial acidity of the setting cement (less than 2.0 pH) may cause sensitivity during and after cementation. The pH however slowly rises to 5.9 within 24 h and is neutral (pH 7.0) by 48 h (Kendzoir and Leinfelder 1976). Zinc phosphate cements have been used successfully in all-metal and metal-supported restorations with very good mechanical retention (parallel walls, more than 4 mm of tooth height, good bulk of the remaining tooth structure). These cements however are not recommended for use in ceramic crowns and composite crowns because of their inferior compressive and flexural strength.

The disadvantages of zinc phosphate cements far outweigh their advantages. They are soluble in oral fluids; they discolor and have weak physical and mechanical properties. Although they can still be found in the dental market, their use in dentistry has become very limited.

1.2.2   Polycarboxylate Cements

Invented in 1968, the polycarboxylate cements use the same powder, zinc oxide, found in the zinc phosphate cements. The liquid however is replaced by a polyacrylic acid solution to improve its resistance to solubility in oral fluids. Because of the polyacrylic acid molecules, there is some form of chemical adhesion to the tooth structure. The polycarboxylates are the first cements to show chemical adhesion to the tooth (Burgess and Ghumann 2011). However, these cements have difficult handling, are tacky, and may be too viscous which makes seating of the restoration difficult.

The main application of polycarboxylate cements today is for the cementation of long-term provisional restorations.

1.2.3   Glass Ionomer Cements

These cements have two main advantages: (1) it offers some degree of chemical adhesion due to its polycarboxylic acid component (the liquid), and (2) it releases fluoride, which is from the fluoro-aluminosilicate glass component (the powder).

However, the adhesive property of the glass ionomer cements is far weaker than those of resin cements. Thus, they are still classified as luting cements.

Glass ionomer cements undergo expansion, an average of 1.7–1.8 % during setting (ADA Professional Product Review 2006). They also expand when they absorb fluids. This property can both be advantageous and disadvantageous. The expansion of glass ionomer cements as they set can contribute to a snugger fit of metal crowns and metal posts. However, this expansion can cause crazing of ceramic crowns as it transmits undue stress to the internal surface of the ceramic restoration.

As glass ionomer cements are soluble to oral fluids and are sensitive to dehydration during its initial set stage, it is recommended to protect the setting cement with a coat of varnish, petroleum jelly, or resin to prevent fluid contamination and desiccation especially on the critical margins. When glass ionomer cement is used for cementation, care should be taken not to dry or dessicate the tooth as this will result to lower bond strengths and postoperative sensitivity (Rosensteil and Rashid 2003).

With these advantages and disadvantages, the use of glass ionomer cements for luting is limited to cementation of indirect restorations with metal subsurfaces. Their retention rates are comparable to zinc phosphate cements.

1.2.4   Resin-Modified Glass Ionomer Cements (Hybrid Cements)

The resin-modified glass ionomer cements were developed to improve on the weaknesses of conventional glass ionomers. The improvements made include substituting part of the polyacrylic acid liquid with hydrophilic methacrylate monomers resulting in higher compressive and tensile strength and less solubility to oral fluids. The adhesive properties and fluoride release of the resin-modified glass ionomer cements are similar to the conventional glass ionomers. It should be noted however that fluoride release in cements is not of much significance as fluoride release depends mainly on the surface area that is exposed to the oral environment. Cements usually have a film thickness of 40–50 μm, which is not enough surface area for significant fluoride release (ADA Professional Product Review 2006).

RMGIs are primarily used for cementation of metal and metal-based restorations (crowns, bridges, inlays/onlays) and orthodontic brackets. They can also be used for the cementation of zirconia and alumina-based ceramics as well as lithium disilicate pressed and milled (CAD/CAM) inlays and onlays. RMGIs still however exhibit hygroscopic expansion upon absorption of fluid and thus cannot be used for the cementation of low-strength all-ceramic crowns and veneers as this may cause clinical fractures.

Although RMGIs have more clinical application than the conventional glass ionomers and zinc phosphates because of their improved properties, they do not have enough bond strengths to retain restorations with poor retention forms such as short clinical crowns and preparations with too much taper and veneers (Table 1.1).

Table 1.1 Conventional cements and representative brands

Cement type	Representative brands
Zinc phosphate	DeTrey Zinc Improved (Dentsply Caulk)
	Fleck's Zinc (Mizzy, Pearson Lab)
	Hy-Bond (Shofu)
	Modern Tenacin (Dentsply Caulk)
Zinc polycarboxylate	Durelon (3 M Espe)
	Shofu Polycarboxylate (Shofu)
	Tylok ®Plus//Poly-F Plus (Dentsply Caulk)
	Durelon Maxicap (3 M Espe)
Conventional glass ionomer	Ketac Cem (3 M Espe)
	Fuji I (GC America)
	Aqua Meron (Voco)
	Meron AC (Voco)
	Riva Luting (SDI)
	GlassLute (Pulpdent)
	CX-Plus (Shofu)
Resin-modified glass ionomer// hybrid cements	FujiCEM (GC America)
	Fuji PLUS (GC)
	RelyX Plus Luting Cement (3 M Espe)
	Riva Luting Plus (SDI Ltd)

1.3   Bonding Cements: The Resin Cements

Bonding cements are more commonly known as resin cements. They have the property to adhere to both the internal surface of the restoration and the tooth structure. The adhesion mechanism of earlier resin cements was mostly micromechanical, but newer cements especially those containing self-etch primers and acidic monomers have been shown to bond chemically to the tooth structure and restoration as well.

Because of their high bond strengths to the tooth structure, the resin cements provide more retention than conventional luting cements. However, they require multiple steps, are difficult to clean up, and are more technique sensitive than conventional cements.

The succeeding chapters will discuss in detail the resin cements.

1.4   Choosing the Right Cement (Luting or Bonding?)

The decision on what cement to use depends mainly on two factors:

I. The restoration material
   The most critical factor in the choice of the cement is the strength of the restoration material. The weaker the material, the stronger should be the cement. Cements that merely lute and do not bond keep the applied forces concentrated

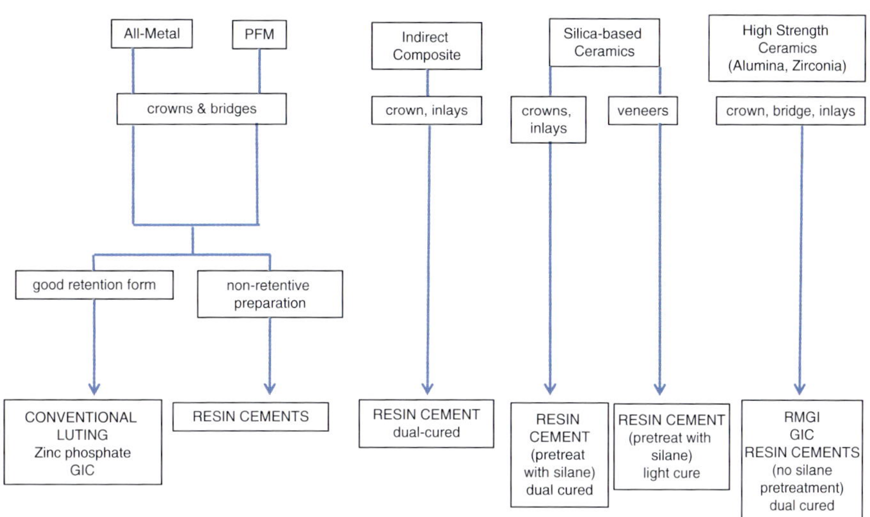

Fig. 1.1 Decision tree on the choice of cement (luting or bonding)

at the tooth-restoration interface; bonded cements dissipate forces applied to the restoration away from the tooth-restoration interface (Chun and White 1999). The cement by being adhesive, in a way, supports the weak restoration. Restorations that are made of metal or have a metal substructure are very strong and alumina and zirconia ceramics have high strength values and do not necessarily need bonding cements. Silica-based ceramics and laboratory composites are weak and thus should be bonded.

II. The amount of retention needed (preparation form, tapers, length of crown/walls)

Preparations with a taper less than 12° and with adequate height (4 mm at least) are considered retentive and do not need to be bonded. The more a preparation becomes non-retentive, the more is the need for bonded cements (Fig. 1.1).

References

ADA Professional Product Review (2006) Dual cure resin-based cements: expert panel discussion. Volume 1(Issue 2 (online)) www.ada.org/goto/ppr

Burgess J, Ghuman T (2011) A practical guide to the use of luting cements – a peer reviewed publication http://www.ineedce.com/courses/1526/PDF/APredictableGuide.pdf. Accessed 12 Feb 2012

Chun LZ, White SN (1999) Mechanical properties of dental luting cements. J Prosthet Dent 81:597–609

Kendzoir GM, Leinfelder KF (1976) Characteristics of zinc phosphate cements mixed at sub-zero temperatures. J Dent Res 55(Special Issue B):B95 [Abstract no. 134]

Rosensteil SF, Rashid RG (2003) Post cementation hypersensitivity: scientific data versus dentists' perceptions. J Prosthodont 12:73

Resin Cements: Factors Affecting Clinical Performance

2

2.1 Introduction

The resin cements are the newest type of cements for indirect restorations, and they have the ability to bond to the tooth structure and the internal surface of the restoration. Resin cements are composed of the same basic component as the composite restorative material but with lower concentration of filler particles (Simon and Darnell 2012). These cements have higher compressive, flexural, and tensile strength than the conventional cements and can be used for almost any type of restoration and restoration material. These cements however are more complex than the conventional cements and are highly technique sensitive.

To maximize the properties of resin cements, a clear understanding of the factors that affect its clinical performance is of paramount importance. These factors are interrelated. The most important factor affecting the success of resin cements is the bond strength of the resin cement. Bond strength in turn is affected by pretreatment procedures, the depth of cure and degree of polymerization of the resin cement, and incompatibilities between the adhesive resin and the resin cement. Factors that may affect polymerization include cement film thickness, opacity, and translucency of both the cement and restoration and shade of the restoration. A properly cured resin cement will exhibit high compressive and flexural strengths, properties that enhance bond strength. Properly cured resin cements are also virtually insoluble to oral fluids. The mode of delivery and method of mixing the resin cement are also factors that may affect the overall clinical performance of the resin cement.

Understanding how all these factors are interrelated will minimize errors and enhance the longevity of bonded indirect restorations. This is intelligent cementation.

© Springer-Verlag Berlin Heidelberg 2015
M. Sunico-Segarra, A. Segarra, *A Practical Clinical Guide to Resin Cements*,
DOI 10.1007/978-3-662-43842-8_2

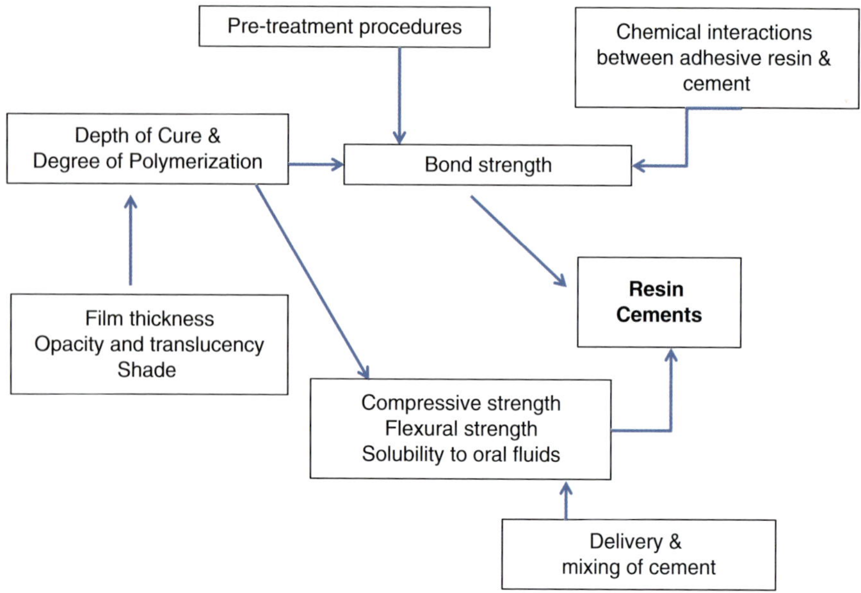

Fig. 2.1 Factors affecting the clinical performance of resin cements

2.2   Pretreatments Prior to the Cementation Procedure

The resin cement bonds the underlying tooth structure to the internal surface of the restoration. Regardless of the type of resin cement, a bond should exist between the dentin and the cement (tooth-cement interface) and between the cement and the internal surface of the restoration (cement-restoration interface) (Fig. 2.1). For these bonds to form, the tooth and the internal surface of the restoration should be pretreated.

2.2.1   Pretreatment of Tooth Structure

Resin cements mainly adhere to the tooth structure through micromechanical retention. To achieve this micromechanical retention, the usual adhesive steps of etching, priming, and bonding should be performed on the enamel and dentin to form a stable hybrid layer. Most resin cement systems come with their proprietary adhesives to avoid incompatibilities between adhesives and cements. Some cements use etch-and-rinse adhesive systems (etch-and-rinse or total etch resin cements), while other cements use adhesives containing self-etch primers (self-etch resin cements). Newer resin cements, the so-called self-adhesive resin cements, have their monomers and adhesives incorporated in the cement itself eliminating the need for pretreatment procedures. As cements adhere to tooth structure through resin bonding, care should be taken that the bonding substrates are clean and free from fluid contamination.

2.2.2 Pretreatment of the Internal Surface of the Restoration

The cement serves as a bridge between the tooth and the restoration. While tooth bonding procedures ensure that the cement adheres well to the tooth, pretreatment of the internal surface of the restoration ensures that the cement will adhere to the restoration as well. A good adhesion to the internal surface of the restoration requires (1) roughening of the internal surface of the restoration to increase the surface area for bonding and (2) increasing the wettability of the cement to the restoration and forming chemical bonds between the ceramic, the fillers, and the cement. Depending on the restoration material, the first procedure is done through air abrasion, sandblasting, or etching with a hydrofluoric acid (for ceramic and composite restorations) or application of an alloy primer (for restorations with a metal subsurface).

The second procedure is achieved by applying a silanating agent on the etched porcelain or composite. The silane makes the ceramic chemically adhere to the resin cement through covalent and hydrogen bonds (Horn 1983). Silanating the internal surface of indirect composite restorations ensures that the fillers of the composite react and adhere with the resin cement (Calamia and Simonsen 1985).

As restoration pretreatments differ from material to material, knowledge of the different types of tooth-colored materials (composites and ceramics) used in dentistry can simplify pretreatment procedures for tooth-colored indirect restorations.

2.3 Classification of Dental Ceramics

There are different ways of classifying ceramics or different terms for different types of ceramics. To simplify it, dental ceramics can be classified into two broad groups based on their composition: the *silica-based ceramics* and the *non-silica-based ceramics* (Blatz and Kern 2003). Since the physical and mechanical properties of ceramics depend mainly on their composition, silica-based ceramics are also referred to as low-to-moderate-strength ceramics, and non-silica-based ceramics are the high-strength ceramics. Based on their structural component and phases, silica-based ceramics are also called glass-ceramic systems, and non-silica-based ceramics are called polycrystalline ceramics. The silica-based ceramics are further classified into feldspathic porcelains, leucite-reinforced ceramics, and lithium disilicate ceramics (Table 2.1).

2.3.1 Pretreatment for Ceramics Based on Their Classification

Dental ceramics, because of their differences in composition and phases, therefore require different pretreatment procedures. *Silica-based ceramics* will require either etching with hydrofluoric acid or sandblasting and subsequent silanization to improve adhesion to the resin cement.

Hydrofluoric acids (HF) roughen the internal surface of the restoration. They are available in varying concentrations from 2.5 to 10 %, and etching time is usually 2–3 min (Chen et al. 1998). Etching ceramic with hydrofluoric acid renders

Table 2.1 Classification of dental ceramics

Classification	Subtypes	Represenatative brands	Flexural strength	Main feature	Indications
Silica-based ceramics (aka: glass-ceramic systems; low-moderate strength ceramics; 1st generation ceramics ceramics	Feldspathic porcelain (aka veneering porcelain)	CEREC Blocs, Eris, Kiss, Classic, LavaCeram, Creation	65–120 MPa	High translucency, very esthetic	Veneers
					As a veneering layer for high strength core ceramics
					Should not be used when there is discoloration or masking is an issue
	Leucite-reinforced ceramic	IPS Empress	120–140 MPa	Highly esthetic	Anterior crowns
					Inlays and onlays
				Leucite crystals act as crack deflectors to increase resistance to crack propagation	As a layering porcelain on high strength ceramic cores
	Lithium disilicate	E-max	300–400 MPa	High strength with good esthetic	Vaneers
					Inlays and onlays
					Posterior crowns
					3-unit bridges (anterior and premolar region)
Non-silica based ceramics (high-strength polycrystalline ceramics)	Alumina	Porcera	650 MPa	High strength	Inlays and onlays
					Posterior crowns
					3-unit bridges
	Zirconia	Lava	800–1,500 MPa	Superior strength	Anterior and posterior crowns
		Cercon			Anterior and posterior bridges
		CERE in Lab		Inherent opacity	Endodontically treated teeth
		InCeram Zirconia		*Randomized clinical trials and clinical experience have been controversial regarding long-term survival[a]*	Maryland bridges (bonding might be a problem)
		IPS emaxZirCAD			Implant abutments
		Katana			Inlay bridges
		Procera AllZirkon			Block-out of darkened tooth structure or cores

[a]Manso et al. (2011)

the surface microscopically porous, increases the surface energy resulting in a microretentive surface (Hussain et al. 1979; Suliman et al. 1993). Care should be taken not to over-etch the porcelain with hydrofluoric acid as it can weaken the bond between the ceramic and resin cement. After HF etching, a white residue sometimes forms on the surface of the porcelain. This white residue is a potential contaminant and should be removed prior to silane application. Recommended methods of removing this residue include immersing in an ultrasonic cleaner for 5 min, steam cleaning, or using an alcohol solution (Alex 2008).

Silane-coupling agents, or simply silane, ensure a good bond between the hydroxyl groups of the ceramic and the organic portion of the resin cement. They are available in two forms (Manso et al. 2011): (1) pre-hydrolyzed single-bottle solutions or (2) two-bottle solutions. Silanes have a rather short shelf life and, once exceeded, are virtually ineffective and unusable. Clinically, a milky-colored solution indicates that the silane is well past its expiration date and should be discarded (Blatz and Kern 2003). This is especially true for the two-bottle systems. Unfortunately, since one-bottle silanes are alcoholic, they stay transparent which makes it difficult to gauge whether they are still usable. Clinicians should strictly respect expiration date and follow manufacturer's instructions when using silanes.

The silane is applied on the internal ceramic surface and then air-dried. There is no consensus on the duration of silane application as it may range from 5 min to 2 h. The usual application time is between 60 and 90 s (Anagnostopoulos et al. 1993; Martinlinna et al. 2004; Alex 2008). This application forms the so-called *interphase layer*, which is actually three layers. The *outermost layer* and the *middle layer* are hydrolyzable and can adversely affect adhesion of the ceramic to the resin cement. These two layers should be removed. The innermost layer, closest to the internal surface of the restoration, is a *monolayer*, which is chemically bonded to the silica phase of the ceramic and is actually responsible for adhesion to the resin cement.

The silanated ceramic should appear dull and not shiny. A shiny surface is indicative of excessive silane and can affect the bond of the ceramic to the resin cement. The silanated surface is then air-dried preferably with warm air. This method of drying, together with the contaminants during the try-in procedure, usually removes the hydrolyzable outermost and middle layers (Ishida 1985).

One important thing to remember is that a hydrofluoric acid-etched ceramic is very prone to contamination with oral fluids. The laboratory usually does the hydrofluoric acid etching. During try-in, the hydrofluoric acid-etched ceramic restoration can be contaminated with saliva. One suggestion to prevent contamination is to apply the silanating agent immediately after hydrofluoric acid etching and prior to try-in as the silane renders the etched ceramic hydrophobic and thus more resistant to fluid contamination. Another advantage of silanating prior to try-in is that the try-in procedure removes the hydrolyzable outermost and middle layers of the silane, rendering the internal surface more conducive to bonding with the resin cement (Manso et al. 2011).

Non-silica-based ceramics such as alumina and zirconia have polycrystalline phase and should not be etched as they are highly resistant to chemical attack from HF (Sorensen et al. 1991; Valandro et al. 2005; Ozcan and Vallitu 2003) or silanated as it might destroy the crystalline structure and weaken the material. Other studies find no improvement in adhesion when alumina and zirconia are etched and silanated prior to cementation. This explains why achieving high and durable bond strengths to alumina and zirconia ceramics is difficult.

The preferred pretreatments for *alumina or aluminum oxide ceramics* include (1) airborne abrasion with 50–110 μm aluminum oxide particles at 2.5 bars, (2) use of an MDP-containing resin cement (Panavia 21, Kuraray, Japan; Single Bond Universal (3 M Espe, Germany)), or (3) silicoating through tribochemical surface treatment (Rocatec, 3 M Espe, Germany) followed by application of a conventional bis-GMA resin cement (Blatz and Kern 2003; Kern et al. 2009; Kitayama et al. 2010; Yun et al. 2010).

Several surface treatments have been studied to improve bonding with *zirconia ceramics*. These include APA (airborne particle abrasion) or wet hand grinding and tribochemical silicoating. APA or wet grinding roughens the surface of the zirconia which was thought to improve bonding. However, some studies have shown that grinding or sandblasting may create surface defects and sharp cracks that render the zirconia prone to cracking or fracture during function (Zhang et al. 2004). Tribochemical silicoating was introduced in an attempt to improve bond without compromising the physical and mechanical properties of zirconia (Kern and Thompson 1994; 1995). In tribochemical silicoating, the internal surface of the zirconia is air abraded with aluminum trioxide particles with silica to coat the zirconia with silica aluminum. This renders the internal surface of the restoration chemically adhere to the resin cement. Studies done on tribochemical silicoating however showed decreased bond strengths with resin cements during aging and thermocycling (Kern and Wegner 1998; Wegner and Kern 2000; Ozcan and Vallitu 2003).

Resin cements and primers containing the acidic monomer 10-MDP are the recommended cements for zirconia ceramics as MDP can chemically bond with zirconia (Tanaka et al. 2008; Oyague et al. 2009). Examples of such cements and primers are Panavia F 2.0, SE Bond, SA Luting Cement (Kuraray, Osaka, Japan) and the newer Scotchbond Universal adhesive (3 M Espe, Germany). Aside from these 10 MDP-containing primers, primers such as Metal/Zirconia Primer (Ivoclar), Z-Primer (Bisco), and AZ Primer (Shofu) which contain phosphoric acid monomers can also be used to promote the adhesion of alumina and zirconia due to chemical bond formation (Kern et al. 2009; Kitayama et al. 2010).

Indirect composite or laboratory composites were developed in an attempt to improve on the physical and mechanical properties of direct composites as well as facilitate carving of adequate proximal contours and contacts and occlusal anatomy. Indirect composites have microhybrid fillers and are highly filled with less of the organic matrix to minimize polymerization shrinkage (Nandini 2010). This class of composites undergoes secondary curing either by heat polymerization or high-intensity light polymerization. Secondary curing has been found to decrease bonding of the restoration to the resin cement as secondary curing leaves no available monomer for subsequent bonding to resin cements (Kildal and Ruyter 1994). Suggested pretreatments for indirect composites include sandblasting followed by phosphoric acid etching the internal surface of the restoration. The sandblasting roughens the internal surface, while phosphoric acid etching cleans the sandblasted surface of debris (Jivraj et al. 2006). Other authors recommend sandblasting followed by application of a silane (Soares et al. 2005) (Table 2.2).

Table 2.2 Surface treatments for the different types of porcelain and laboratory composites

Type of ceramic	Representative brands	Pre-treatment Roughening of internal surface	Silane
Feldspathic porcelain	CEREC Blocs, Eris, Kiss, Classic, LavaCeram, Creation	HF acid 2.5–10 % for 2–3 min or	Apply silane following manufacturer's instructions
Leucite-reinforced ceramic	IPS Empress	Sandblasting/air abrasion or	
Lithium disilicate	IPS E-max	Sandblasting + HF acid etching	
Alumina/aluminum oxide	Procera	1. Airborne particle abrasion (APA) using 50–110 μ AlO_2 at 2.5 bars or	Do not silanate
	In Ceram	2. Use an MDP containing resin cement and primer (Panavia F 2.0, Universal Bond) or	Do not silanate
Zirconia/zirconium oxide	Lava	3. Silicacoating (tribochemical surface treatment)	
	Cercon	4. APA or silicacoating + use an MDP containing resin cement	
	CEREC inLab InCeram Zirconia IPS emaxZirCAD Katana Procera AllZirkon	5.Use a phosphoric acid monomer containing primer (Z-Primer, Metal/Zirconia Primer, AZ Primer)	
Indirect composites (laboratory composites)	Artglass, Belleglass HP, Sinfony, SR Adoro, Sculpture Plus, Tescera, Ceramage	Sandblasting with AlO_2 for 10 s OR Sandblasting followed by phosphoric acid etching	Apply silane No need for silane

2.4   Physical and Mechanical Properties of the Resin Cement

The following physical and mechanical properties directly affect the clinical performance of resin cements (McCabe and Walls 2008):

1. Compressive strength
2. Flexural strength
3. Film thickness
4. Solubility and water sorption

2.4.1 Compressive Strength

Luting cements should have good compressive strength to be able to withstand masticatory forces in the mouth. As resin cements are bonded to both the tooth structure and the restoration, a high compressive strength of the cement also increases the fracture resistance of the restoration, particularly brittle materials such as ceramics. This is particularly true for the first-generation silica-based feldspathic ceramics, which have very low flexural strength (65–120 MPa) (Powers et al. 2013).

2.4.2 Flexural Strength

Flexural strength is that property of a material to withstand bending forces without breaking. In a tooth-cement-restoration assembly, the cement should have adequate flexural strength to be able to transmit the stresses between the tooth and restoration without breaking. This will protect the brittle restorative material. Moreover, the closer the elastic modulus of the cement to that of the dentin, the less will be the stress concentrations at the cement tooth interface and will result to a more durable bond. Resin cements are approximately 20× stronger and 130× tougher in flexure than conventional cements, which make them the material of choice in the cementation of all-ceramic restorations (Chun and White 1999).

2.4.3 Film Thickness and Viscosity

Considerable differences in film thickness occur between resin cements (Varjao et al. 2002). As a rule, luting cements should exhibit low film thickness. A low cement film thickness improves seating of the restoration and decreases marginal discrepancies which in turn will help reduce plaque accumulation, periodontal disease, cement dissolution, and eventual secondary caries formation. Resin cements have been shown to exhibit a somewhat higher film thickness than conventional cements (Yu et al. 1995). Although resin cements are less soluble in oral fluids, which will compensate for this higher film thickness, a high film thickness can prevent proper seating of the restoration. Studies have also shown that increased film thickness can decrease the tensile strength of cast restorations (Scherrer et al. 1994). An increased film thickness of greater than 300 μm has also been shown to cause gradual decrease in fracture strength resulting to cracks (Levine 1989) and lower bond strengths in all-ceramic restorations (Cekic-Nagas et al. 2010). Evidence shows that a lower cement film thickness (less than 50 μm) is more advantageous for all-ceramic restorations (Levine 1989).

According to the American Dental Association (ADA) Specification for luting agents, a film thickness of 25 μm is required for Type I cements and 40 μm for Type II cements. Type I cements because of their low film thickness are recommended for precision restorations such as inlays, while Type II cements are commonly used for fixed partial prostheses. When using cements that fall within the Type II category, a thicker die relief is recommended to compensate for the higher film thickness of the cement (Fusayama et al. 1964).

The film thickness of resin cements can usually be found in the products literature that come with the cement.

2.4.4   Solubility and Water Sorption

Although resin cements are insoluble to oral fluids, being resins, they absorb water. When resin cements absorb water, their flexural strength is decreased (Oysaed and Ruyter 1986). The thicker the cement, the greater will be the decrease in flexural strength (plasticizing effect) which makes the cement unable to dissipate stresses from masticatory function between tooth and restoration. This may result to eventual fracture of the ceramic. It is thus important that resin cement layers be kept to a thin layer to minimize the plasticizing phenomenon or resin cements (Ferracane et al. 1998).

2.5   Bond Strength

Since the function of the resin cement is to retain the restoration through adhesion, adequate bond strengths to the underlying tooth structure are very important. Resin cements are also classified according to mechanism of adhesion. Different types of resin cements will exhibit different bond strengths to enamel and to dentin. The choice of resin cement greatly depends on the degree of retention needed. The more retention is needed (such as short crowns, preparations with too much taper, etc.); cements with higher bond strengths are better.

A more detailed discussion on the bond strengths of the different types of resin cements is included in the next chapter.

2.6   Depth of Cure and Degree of Polymerization

Resin cements can be classified according to mode of polymerization.

2.6.1   Self-Curing Resin Cements

These cements set through chemical reaction and are especially useful in areas that are difficult to reach with light. Examples are metal restorations, porcelain fused to metals, and thick ceramic restorations (Simon and Darnell 2012). These cements contain the tertiary amine benzoyl peroxide that initiates polymerization. The peroxide molecules are the ones responsible for color shift during aging.

2.6.2   Dual-Cured Resin Cements

These cements cure by both light curing and chemical curing, hence the name "dual." These types of cements contain both a self-cured initiator (benzoyl peroxide) and a light-cured initiator (camphoroquinone). The initial set is usually achieved with light curing to quickly seal the gingival margins (Vohra et al. 2013). The self-curing component ensures that the cement will cure underneath restorations that are too thick or too opaque to allow transmission of light through it (Pegoraro et al.

2007). Dual-cured resin cements although they can set through chemical reaction alone still require light curing to achieve a high degree of polymerization.

2.6.3 Light-Cured Resin Cements

These cements set exclusively through light polymerization. The most common photoinitiator is camphoroquinone although some cements may contain a different photoinitiator. Because of this, the clinician should be aware of the type of photoinitiator present in the resin cement as some curing lights may not match the spectrum of absorption of the photoinitiator.

As most, if not all, resin cements have a light curing component, the depth of cure and degree of polymerization is a very important factor to consider. Insufficient polymerization of the resin cement can lead to increased solubility especially at the margins leading to marginal gaps and secondary caries, marginal discoloration, pulpal reactions, and increased fluid absorption which can lead to hygroscopic expansion and changes in color (color shift) due to the unreacted camphoroquinone photoinitiators. Insufficiently polymerized resin cement has decreased hardness, fracture toughness, and wear resistance and can also lead to lower bond strengths (Vohra et al. 2013). Reducing the exposure time for dual-cured and light-cured resin cements to 75 % of that recommended by the manufacturer will likewise increase water sorption (Pearson and Longman 1989).

Several factors affect the depth of cure and degree of polymerization of resin cements (Table 2.3). Factors related to the restoration include restoration thickness, opacity, and shade. Factors related to the resin cement include mode of polymerization (light cured, dual cured), opacity of the cement, film thickness, filler particle size, and filler loading. Factors related to the light source include distance, duration of exposure, light intensity, and wavelength that matches the spectrum of absorption of the cement's photoinitiator.

2.7 Color Shift

Resins that contain the tertiary amine benzoyl peroxide in self-cured and dual-cured resins tend to darken with time. The photoinitiator camphoroquinone in light-cured cements is more color stable. However, the cement should be sufficiently polymerized as unreacted camphoroquinone turns yellow with age. Some resin cements use a different kind of photoinitiator other than the tertiary amines to prevent any form of color shift.

2.8 Chemical Interactions Between the Adhesive Resin and the Cement

Incompatibilities between simplified adhesives and dual-cured resin cements exist, especially for etch-and-rinse single-bottle adhesives and the seventh-generation all-in-one self-etch adhesives. These adhesives are inherently acidic and hydrophilic.

Table 2.3 Factors affecting polymerization of dual-cured and light-cured resin cements

Material-related factors	Thickness of the restoration	For purely light-cured resin cements—thickness should not be >0.8 mm For dual-cured resin cements—linear reduction in hardness as the thickness of the cement increases. Optimum material thickness is 2.0 mm (Pazin et al. 2008)
	Translucency/opacity	More translucent shades, greater degree of polymerization (Llie and Hickel 2008) Feldspathic porcelains are more translucent than other types of ceramics, more efficient polymerization (Borges et al. 2008) Opaque porcelains need longer curing time (twice as long)
	Shade (less effect on polymerization than translucency)	Darker shade of restoration may need longer curing time (twice as long)
Factors related to resin cement	Mode of polymerization (light cured or dual cured)	Dual-cured cements should be light cured to gain initial immediate set—protects the cement on the margin and ensures adequate marginal seal
	Opacity of the cement	More translucent shades have greater polymerization; increase polymerization time for opaque cements
	Film thickness	Type II cements (film thickness of >40 μm) require longer polymerization time
	Filler particle size and filler loading	> filler particle size and higher filler loading =>depth of cure; explains why flowable composites which have very small filler particle size and loading have less depth of cure than resin cements
Factors related to light source	Distance	Should be as close to the restoration as possible; greater distance of restoration from light tip requires increase in curing time
	Intensity of light	No less than 800 mw/cm^3
	Duration of exposure	Follow manufacturer's instruction but longer for opaque materials, opaque cements, darker shade of restoration, and increased distance (twice longer than manufacturer's instructions)
	Wavelength	Most resin cements use camphoroquinone as the photoinitiator—wavelength of light should be from 420 to 500 nm

Incompatibilities occur because the oxygen-inhibited layer of the acidic simplified adhesives reacts with the tertiary amine of the dual-cured resin cement creating a so-called acid dissolution zone that does not completely set and eventually result to poor bonding (Sanares et al. 2001) (Fig. 2.2). Also, as these adhesives are hydrophilic, they are still somewhat permeable even after polymerization, which further compromises the bond (Tay et al. 2002). This incompatibility becomes more significant

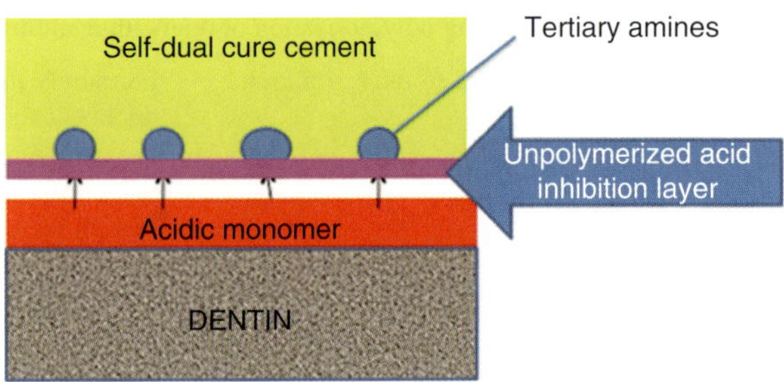

Fig. 2.2 The acid inhibition layer formed when the acidic monomer of simplified adhesives attack the tertiary amine initiator of self- and dual-cured resin cements

when the cement takes harder to cure by light such as in situations where distance from the light is greater, when cementing thick restorations and in the cementation of posts, as it takes more time for the cement to attain complete polymerization allowing for more formation of the acid-inhibited zone (Manso et al. 2011).

To avoid adverse interaction between the adhesive system and the dual-cured cement, three-step etch-prime-bond systems or two-step self-etch systems are recommended (Tay et al. 2003; Carvalho et al. 2005). The application of a separate layer of pure hydrophobic bonding resin forms a barrier between the adhesive's oxygen-inhibited layer and the amine of the resin cement (King et al. 2005). Some resin cements come with a dual-cured activator, which acts as a barrier between the acidic monomer and tertiary amine to prevent incompatibilities. Incompatibilities can also be avoided by using the self-adhesive resin cements instead as they do not require that the tooth be treated first with adhesives prior to cementation (Manso et al. 2011).

References

Alex G (2008) Preparing porcelain surfaces for optimal bonding. Funct Esthet Restor Dent 1:38–46

Anagnostopoulos T, Eliades G, Palaghias G (1993) Composition, reactivity and surface interactions of three dental silane primers. Dent Mater 9:182–190

Blatz MK, Kern M (2003) Resin-ceramic bonding: a review of the literature. J Prosthet Dent 89:268–274

Borges GA, Agarwal P, Miranzi BAS et al (2008) Influence of different ceramics on resin cement Knoop hardness number. Oper Dent 33:622–628

Calamia JR, Simonsen RJ (1985) Effects of coupling agents on bond strength of etched porcelain (Abstract). J Dent Res 64:296 (Special issue)

Carvalho RM, Garcia FC, de Silva SM et al (2005) Adhesive-composite incompatibility, part II. J Esthet Restor Dent 17:191–195

Cekic-Nagas I, Canay S, Sahin E (2010) Bonding of resin core materials to lithium disilicate ceramics: the effect of resin film thickness. Int J Prosthodont 23:469–471

Chen JH, Matsumura H, Atsuta M (1998) Effect of etchant, etching periods on the bond strength of a composite resin to a machinable porcelain. J Dent 23:250–257

Chun LZ, White SN (1999) Mechanical properties of dental luting cements. J Prosthet Dent 81:597–609

Fusayama T, Ide K, Hosada H (1964) Relief of resistance of cement of full cast crowns. J Prosthet Dent 14:95–106

Horn HR (1983) Porcelain laminate veneers bonded to etch enamel. Dent Clin North Am 27:671–684

Hussain MA, Bradford EW, Charlton G (1979) Effect of etching on the strength of aluminous porcelain jacket crowns. BDJ 147:89–90

Ferracane JL, Berge HX, Condon JR (1998) In vitro aging of dental composites in water – effect of degree of conversion, filler volume, and filler/matrix coupling. J Biomed Mater Res 42:465–472

Ishida H (1985) Structural gradient in the silane-coupling agent layers and its influence on the mechanical and physical properties of composites. Plenum Press, New York, pp 25–50

Jivraj SA, Kim TH, Donovan T (2006) Selection of luting agents part 1. CDA Journal 34(2): 149–160

Kern M, Barloi A, Yang B (2009) Surface conditioning influences zirconia ceramic bonding. J Dent Res 88:817–822

Kern M, Thompson VP (1994) Sandblasting and silica coating of a glass-infiltrated alumina ceramic: volume loss, morphology, and changes in the surface composition. J Prosthet Dent 71:453–461

Kern M, Thompson VP (1995) Bonding to glass-infiltrated alumina ceramic: adhesive methods and their durability. J Prosthet Dent 73:240–249

Kern M, Wegner SM (1998) Bonding to zirconia ceramic: adhesion methods and their durability. Dent Mater 14:64–71

Kildal KK, Ruyter JE (1994) How different curing methods affect the degree of conversion of resin based inlay/onlay materials. Acta Odontologica Scand 152(5):315–322

King NM, Tay FR, Pashley DH et al (2005) Conversion o one-step to two-step self-etch adhesives for improved efficacy and extended application. Am J Dent 18:126–134

Kitayama S, Nikaido T, Takahashi R et al (2010) Effect of primer treatment on bonding of resin cements to zirconia ceramic. Dent Mater 26:426–432

Levine WA (1989) An evaluation of the film thickness of resin luting agents. J Prosthet Dent 62:175–178

Llie N, Hickel R (2008) Correlation between ceramics translucency and polymerization efficiency through ceramic. Dent Mater 24:208–214

Manso AP, Silva NR, Bonfante EA et al (2011) Cements and adhesives for all-ceramic restorations. Dent Clin N Am 55:311–332

Martinlinna JP, Lassila LV, Ozcan M et al (2004) An introduction to silanes and their clinical applications in dentistry. Int J Prosthodont 17:155–164

McCabe JF, Walls AW (2008) Applied dental materials, 9th edn. Blackwell, Oxford, UK, pp 274–285

Nandini S (2010) Indirect resin composites J Conserv Dent (serial online) (cited 2013 January 7);13:184–194. Available from: http://www.jcd.org.in/text.asp?2010/13/4/184/73377

Oyague RC, Monticelli F, Toledano M et al (2009) Effect of water aging on microtensile bond strength of dual-cured resin cements to pretreated sintered zirconium oxide ceramics. Dent Mater 25:392–399

Oysaed H, Ruyter IE (1986) Composites for use in posterior teeth: mechanical properties tested under dry and wet conditions. J Biomed Mater Res 20:261–271

Ozcan M, Vallitu PK (2003) Effect of surface conditioning methods on the bond strength of luting cement to ceramics. Dent Mater 19:725–731

Pazin MC, Moraes RR, Goncalves LS et al (2008) Effects of ceramic thickness and curing light on light transmission through leucite-reinforce material and polymerization of dual-cured luting agent. J Oral Sci 50:131–136

Pearson GJ, Longman CM (1989) Water sorption and solubility of resin-based materials following inadequate polymerization by a visible-light curing system. J Oral Rehabil 16:57–61

Pegoraro TA, Da Silva NR, Carvalho RM (2007) Cements for use in esthetic dentistry. Dent Clin North Am 51:187–192

Powers JM, Farah JW, O'Keefe KL et al (2013) Guide to all-ceramic bonding. Available from: http://www.Kuraraydental.com/guides/-item/guide-to-all-ceramic-bonding. Accessed 31 July 2013

Sanares AM, Itthagarun A, King NM et al (2001) Adverse surface interactions between one-bottle light-cured adhesives and chemical-cured composites. Dent Mater 17:542–556

Scherrer SS, de Rijk WG, Belser UC et al (1994) Dent Mater 10:172–177

Simon JF, Darnell LA (2012) Consideration for proper selection of dental cements. Compend Contin Educ Dent 33:28–36

Soares CJ, Soares PV, Pereira JC, Fonesca RB (2005) Surface treatment protocols in the cementation process of ceramic and laboratory processed composite restorations. A literature review. J Esthet Restor Dent 17:24–35

Sorensen JA, Engelman MJ, Torres TJ et al (1991) Shear bond strength of composite resin to porcelain. Int J Prosthodont 4:17–23

Suliman AH, Swift EJ Jr, Perdiago J (1993) Effects of surface treatment and bonding agents on bond strength of composite resin to porcelain. J Prosthet Dent 70:118–120

Tanaka R, Fujishima A, Shibata Y et al (2008) Cooperation of phosphate monomer and silica modification on zirconia. J Dent Res 87:666–670

Tay FR, Pashley DH, Suh BI et al (2002) Single-step adhesives are permeable membranes. J Dent 30:371–382

Tay FR, Bl S, Pashley DH et al (2003) Factors contributing to the incompatibility between simplified-step adhesives and self-cured or dual-cured composites. Part II. Single-bottle, total-etch adhesive. J Adhes Dent 5:91–105

Valandro LF, Della Bona A, Antonio Bottino M et al (2005) The effect of ceramic surface treatment on bonding to densely sintered alumina ceramic. J Prosthet Dent 93:253–259

Varjão FM, Segalla JCM, Beloti AM et al (2002) Study on film thickness of four resin cements. Rev Odontol UNESP São Paulo 31:171–177

Vohra F, Al-Rifaiy M, Al Aqhtani M (2013) Factors affecting resin polymerization of bonded all ceramic restorations. Review of literature. J Dow Uni Health Sci Karachi 7:80–86

Wegner SM, Kern M (2000) Long-term resin bond strength to zirconia ceramic. J Adhes Dent 2:139–147

Yu Z et al (1995) Effect of dynamic loading methods on cement film thickness in vitro. J Prosthodont 4(4):252–255

Yun JY, Ha SR, Lee JB et al (2010) Effect of sandblasting and various metal primers on the shear bond strength of resin cement to Y-TZP ceramic. Dent Mater 26:650–658

Zhang Y, Lawn BR, Rekow ED et al (2004) Effect of sandblasting on the long term performance of dental ceramics. J Biomed Mater Res B Appl Biomater 71:381–386

Part II

Clinical Aspects of Resin Cements

Classification of Resin Cements

3

3.1 Introduction

Resin cements are the newest types of cements used to lute and bond indirect restorations. They have higher compressive, tensile, and flexural strength and wear resistance compared to the conventional luting cements. They come in different shades and are virtually insoluble in oral fluids providing better marginal seal than any other cement types. These categories of cements can be used for all types of restorative materials (porcelain, metal, porcelain fused to metal, laboratory composites).

Resin cements should bond both to the tooth structure and the internal surface of the restoration. In the previous chapter, the bonding mechanism of the resin cement to the internal surface of the restoration was discussed in detail. This chapter focuses mainly on the adhesion of the resin cement to the tooth surface.

In current clinical practice, there are three available resin cements in the market classified according to their adhesive characteristics. These are the etch-and-rinse resin cements, also called total-etch cements, the self-etch resin cements, and the self-adhesive resin cements (Fig. 3.1). Numerous terminologies pertaining to these three types of cements can be found in books and journals, which add to the confusion in classification. Some authors call the etch-and-rinse cements and self-etch cements conventional resin cements (CR cements) as they require adhesive pretreatment of the tooth surface, i.e., etching, priming, and bonding. The self-adhesive resin cements are sometimes referred to as simply adhesive resin cements (AR) or true adhesive cements as they can bond to the tooth surface on their own without the need for prior etching and bonding.

Generally, the etch and rinse resin cements yield the highest bond strengths to enamel, while self-etch resin cements show higher bond strengths to dentin. Self-adhesive resin cements have lower bond strengths than the total etch and self-etch resin cements (Sanvin and de Rijk 2006).

© Springer-Verlag Berlin Heidelberg 2015
M. Sunico-Segarra, A. Segarra, *A Practical Clinical Guide to Resin Cements*,
DOI 10.1007/978-3-662-43842-8_3

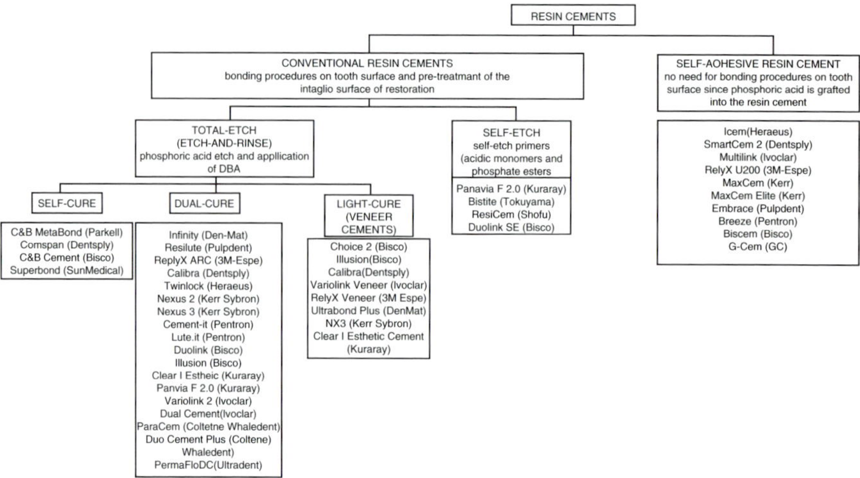

Fig. 3.1 Classification of resin cements and some representative brands

3.2 The Etch-and-Rinse Cements (Total-Etch Cements)

3.2.1 Description

These cements are those that use etch-and-rinse or total-etch adhesives. The enamel and dentin surface is etched with 36–37 % phosphoric acid followed by an application of a single layer of the single-bottle self-priming adhesive (dentin-bonding agent or DBA) prior to cementation with the resin cement. These cements, depending on the brand, can be self-cured, dual cured, or light cured. The veneer cements are included in this category.

3.2.2 Technical and Clinical Considerations

Since etch-and-rinse cements involve etching the enamel and dentin with phosphoric acid, they yield the highest bond strengths to the enamel among all resin cements. When used properly, they yield high bond strengths to dentin (Casseli and Martins 2006). Like all resins which bond using etch-and-rinse adhesives, however, these cements require the most number of steps and are more technique sensitive than the other types of resin cements (Burgess et al. 2010). The clinical success of these cements is greatly affected by operator factors. Tooth isolation is of paramount importance with these cements. Some recommend that they be best used for easy to isolate areas in the mouth, the anterior segment (ADA Expert Panel 2006). Another concern with this type of cement is postoperative sensitivity that occurs if the opened dentinal tubules from acid etching are not well sealed (Christensen 2007). Additionally, dentin is less calcified than the enamel, and prolonged phosphoric acid

Table 3.1 Advantages and disadvantages of etch-and-rinse resin cements

Advantages	Disadvantages
Higher bond strengths to the enamel and other highly calcified tooth structures (sclerotic dentin, fluorosed enamel, etc.)	Multistep
High bond strength to dentin if used properly, strict attention to details	Technique sensitive
Usually come in many shades—good shade matching	Possibility of postoperative sensitivity if not used properly on dentin surfaces

etching can lead to decrease in bond strengths. When using these cements, therefore, care should be taken not to etch the dentin for more than 20 s to prevent postoperative sensitivity. There is also concern about the incompatibilities between the acidic dentin-bonding agent used in conjunction with these cements and the amine initiators of some self- and dual-cured cements in this category. Some authors recommend the additional application of a self-cured activator over the adhesive layer prior to cementation to avoid such incompatibilities (King et al. 2005).

In summary, the keys to successful cementation and preventing postoperative sensitivity with etch-and-rinse resin cements are as follows:

1. Do not overdry the tooth, especially after etching. The surface should appear glossy.
2. Limit etching time to 15 s only on dentin.
3. Ensure adequate sealing of the dentinal tubules through proper application of the dentin-bonding agent.
4. Ensure proper tooth isolation, preferably with a rubber dam.
5. When using self- or dual-cured resin cement, use a self-cured activator to prevent incompatibilities between the amine initiator of the cement and the acidic DBA.

3.2.3   Indications

Factoring in all the advantages and disadvantages of resin cements (Table 3.1), these cements are recommended for the following:

1. Restorations where the predominant tooth structure present is the enamel such as in the case of veneers.
2. Preparations on highly calcified tooth structures (fluorosis, sclerotic dentin, arrested dentin).
3. Enamel margins of inlays and onlays (using the selective etch technique). The selective etch technique involves etching with phosphoric acid the enamel margins only for 20 s. The etchant is then washed off and the tooth dried, and a self-etch adhesive is then applied on both the enamel and dentin.

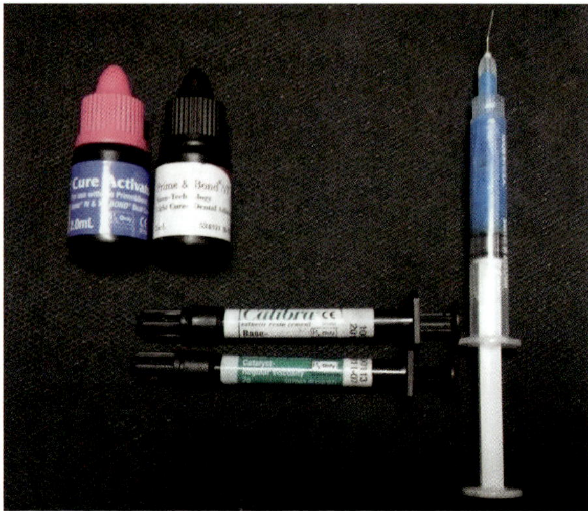

Fig. 3.2 Example of a total-etch resin cement, Calibra (Dentsply Caulk). The starter kit comes with a phosphoric acid etchant, a one-bottle DBS, a self-cure activator, and base and catalyst pastes

4. Cementation of low-strength ceramics (feldspathic porcelains) as high bond strengths can strengthen the low-strength ceramic.
5. Maryland bridges.

3.2.4 Manipulation

Total-etch resin cements either come in two-paste systems or paste-powder systems and with their corresponding etchant and single-bottle dentin-bonding agents. A self-cured activator is also included with the kit. The dual-cured activator serves as a barrier between the acidic single-bottle DBA and the amines of the dual-cured or self-cured resin cement. The porcelain etchant (HF acid) and silane used for pretreatment of the ceramics and laboratory composites are sold separately (Fig. 3.2).

Some total-etch resin cements can be completely self-cured. Examples are C&B Metabond (Parkell), Comspan (Dentsply), C&B Cement (Bisco), and Superbond C&B (Sun Medical). These cements are not recommended for veneers as there is limited working time to properly fit and seat the veneers due to their self-curing mode. Furthermore, because of their self-cured mechanism, they contain an amine initiator which has a yellowing effect during aging causing color shift. This yellowing can show through the thin veneer material and can compromise esthetics (Fig. 3.3).

Total-etch dual-cured resin cements come in two-paste systems (base paste and catalyst paste). When the base and catalyst pastes are mixed together, they set by both self- and light-cured mechanisms. To make the cement set only by light curing, such as in the case of veneer cementation, only the base paste is used. Examples of these cements are Calibra (Dentsply) and Variolink (Ivoclar Vivadent).

Light-cured resin cements specifically veneer or aesthetic cements come in a single syringe and can only polymerize with the application of light. These cements come in different shades (Fig. 3.4).

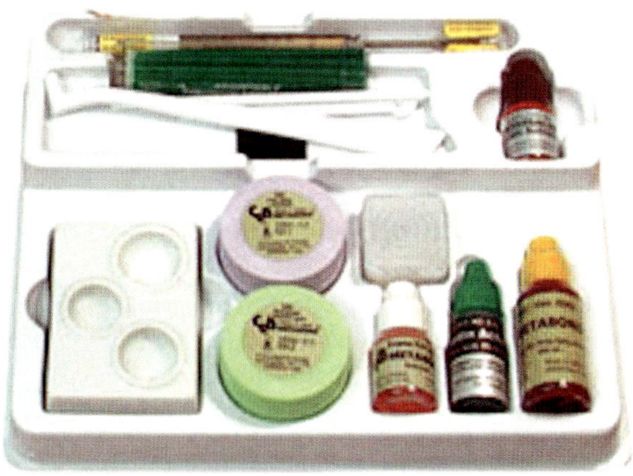

Fig. 3.3 An example of a self-cured total-etch resin cement, C&B Metabond (Parkell)

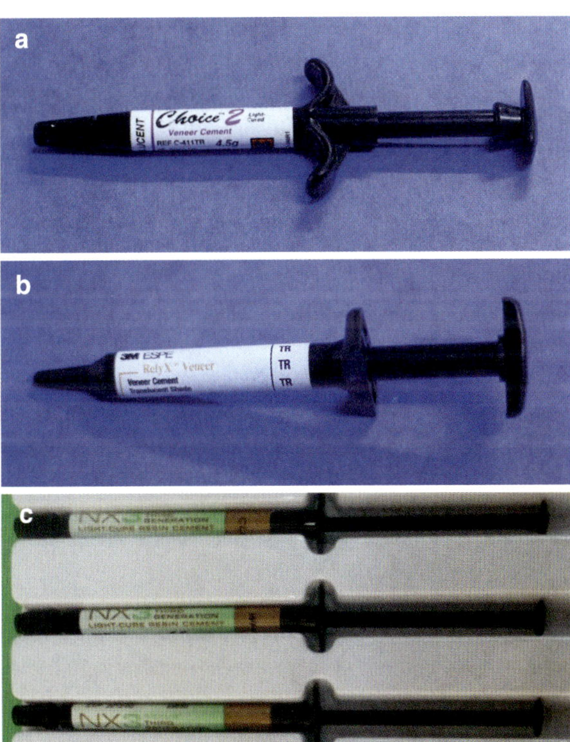

Fig. 3.4 Examples of veneer cements. (**a**) Choice 2 (Bisco), (**b**) RelyX Veneer (3M Espe), and (**c**) Nexus 2 (Kerr)

3.3   The Self-Etch Resin Cements

3.3.1   Description

These cements are simpler to use as phosphoric acid etching is eliminated. Instead, the etchant, composed of acidic monomers and phosphate esters, is combined with the primer, thus the name self-etch primers. Common acidic monomers include 10-MDP found in Panavia F (Kuraray), 4-META, and GPDM. The adhesive to pretreat the tooth surface for most self-etch resin cements comes in two bottles, which are dispensed in equal amounts and are thoroughly mixed. These cements are mostly dual cured. Because of its ease of use due to the elimination of phosphoric acid etching step, most clinicians prefer the self-etch resin cements to the total-etch cements.

3.3.2 Clinical and Technical Considerations

Data shows that self-etch resin cements yield comparable, if not higher dentin bond strengths to total-etch resin cements. Generally, however, bond strengths to the enamel are weaker than that of total-etch systems. They bond better to the dentin than to the enamel. This can be attributed to the weaker etchants in self-priming systems (acidic monomer vs. phosphoric acid).

An advantage of self-etch resin cements is that during the entire adhesive procedure, the smear layer is not removed, preventing the inflow and outflow of fluid from the dentinal tubules. Postoperative dentistry is thus lessened. Also, there is less risk of over-etching the dentin as the acid is weaker, decalcification of the dentin is less, and a thinner but well-infiltrated hybrid layer is formed. This explains why dentin bonds for self-etch resin cements are higher than that of total-etch cements in some studies.

A common step usually ignored in self-etch adhesives is the air-drying after adhesive application. The adhesive should be air-dried for about 5–10 s as drying removes the residual acidic hydrogen ions and ethanol. If not air-dried, the hydrogen and ethanol remain in the set adhesive layer. The residual hydrogen will cause continuous etching, while the ethanol can cause hydrolysis of the bonds, which is clinically seen as brownish discoloration on the margins. Manufacturer's instructions during adhesive application and adhesive cementation should always be followed.

Self-etch resin cements are usually stored under refrigeration and away from sunlight as heat degrades the acidic monomers.

3.3.3 Indications (Table 3.2)

Resin cements can be used for any type of restoration material (metal, ceramic, and composite). However, taking into consideration all their advantages and disadvantages, self-etch resin cements are specifically best for the following situations:

1. Crowns and bridges with a lot of healthy dentin exposed
2. When retention is compromised:
    (a) Short crowns with less than 4 mm height
    (b) Crown tapers of more than 14°
3. Crowns and other fixed prostheses that have repeatedly come off
4. Inlays and onlays, especially those with deep cavities and few walls remaining

Table 3.2 Advantages and disadvantages of self-etch resin cements

Advantages	Disadvantages
Good bond strength to the dentin	Relatively weaker bonds to the enamel and highly calcified tooth structures
Ease of use (no need for a separate phosphoric acid etching step, rinsing and drying)	May still cause postoperative sensitivity if adhesive is not air-dried
Less risk of over-etching the dentin	Most self-etch resin cements need refrigeration as acidic monomers degrade with heat
Less risk of postoperative sensitivity, however	Less available shades compared to total-etch resin cements

3.3.4   Manipulation

Most self-etch resin cements come in two-paste systems and are dual cured (Fig. 3.4). These cements are very specific as to the type of adhesive that should be used in conjunction with them to avoid any incompatibilities (Fig. 3.5).

The self-etch adhesive usually comes in two bottles. Equal amounts of each liquid are dispensed in a mixing well and mixed thoroughly for 5–10 s to ensure good chemical reaction (Fig. 3.6).

The adhesive is then applied on the bonding surfaces of the tooth using a light rubbing motion for 20 s or as per manufacturer's instructions. The adhesive is lightly air-dried with oil-free air for a minimum of 20 s. The air-drying removes the solvents and excess water leaving a thin but well-infiltrated hybrid layer. The adhesive is then light cured to stabilize the hybrid layer.

Pastes A and B of the resin cement are dispensed in equal amounts on a mixing pad. Some self-etch resin cements come in twist tubes where each twist of the tube is marked by a line to ensure that exact amounts of base and catalyst pastes are dispensed (Fig. 3.7).

Some self-etch resin cements come in an autodispenser (Fig. 3.8) to ensure that equal amounts of cements are dispensed.

The pastes are then mixed with a plastic spatula using folding strokes to ensure that there are no air bubbles entrapped (Fig. 3.9).

3.4   Self-Adhesive Resin Cements

3.4.1   Description

The self-adhesive resin cements are the newest in this category. Also called one-component "universal adhesive cements," these cements do not require a separate bonding procedure on the tooth as phosphoric acid is grafted in the resin in the form of phosphoric esters. The phosphoric acid reacts with the composite fillers forming

Fig. 3.5 Examples of self-etch resin cements (from top: **a**) Panavia F 2.0 (Kuraray); (**b**) ResiCem (Shofu); (**c**) Bistite (Tokuyama). They are two-paste systems, and the corresponding adhesive comes in two or three bottles (primers A and B). An oxygen barrier is usually included in the kit

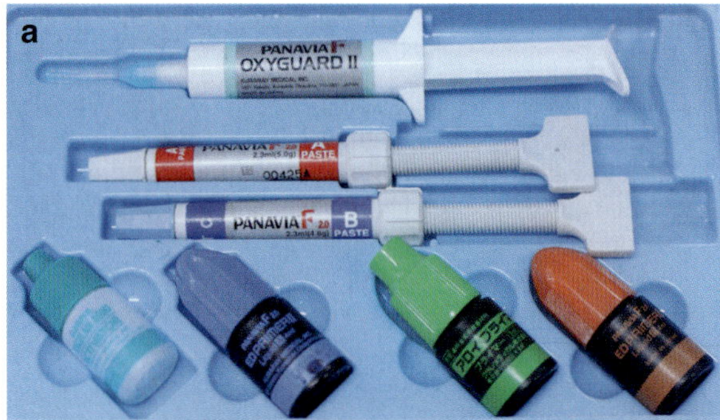

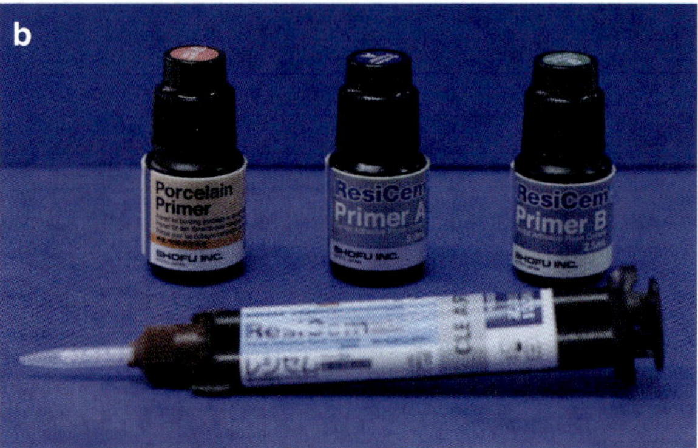

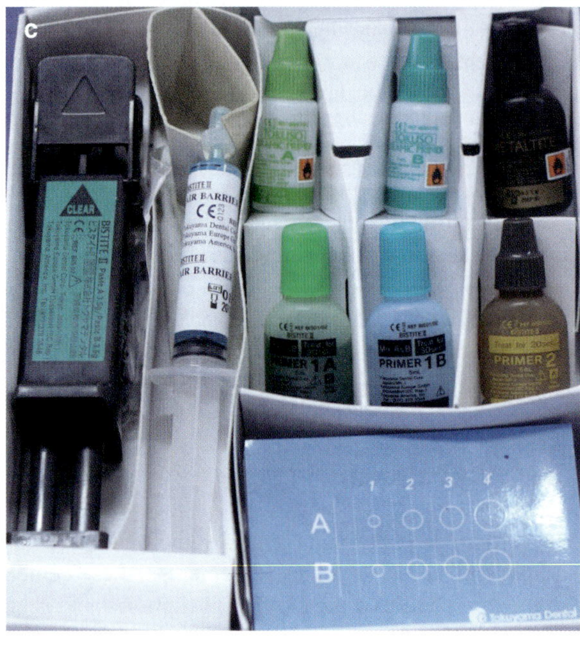

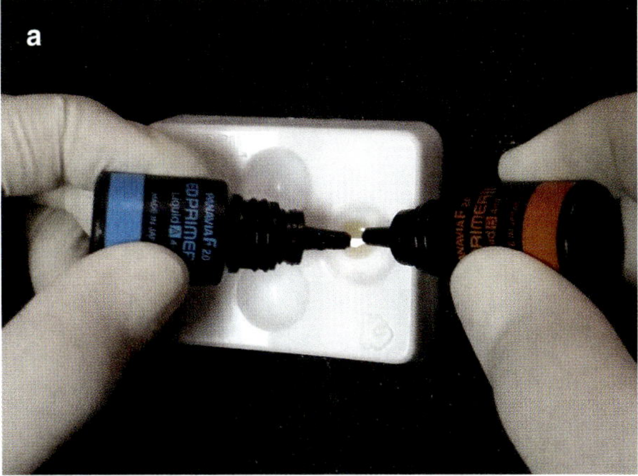

Fig. 3.6 (**a**) Dispensing equal amounts of primers A and B and (**b**) mixing them thoroughly

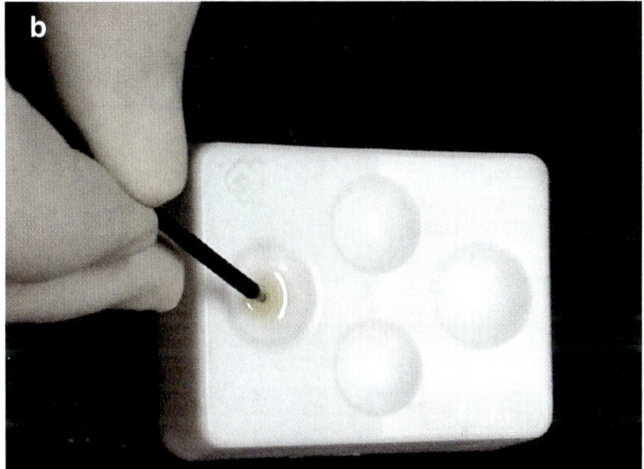

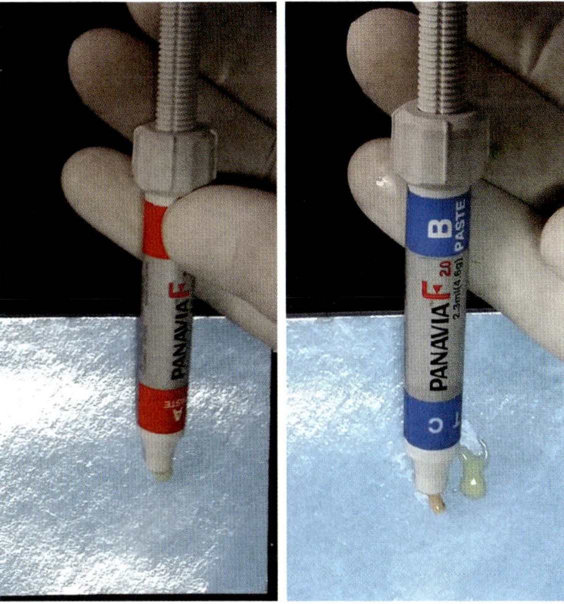

Fig. 3.7 Twist tubes with line indicating the amount of paste dispensed

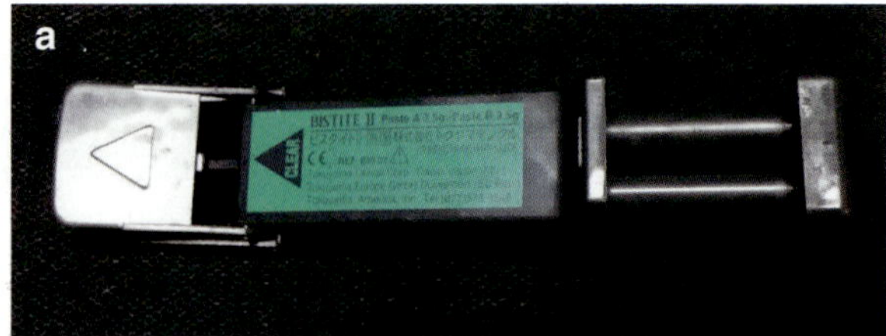

Fig. 3.8 Autodispensers for (**a**) Bistite (Tokuyama) and (**b**) ResiCem (Shofu), with an automixing tip

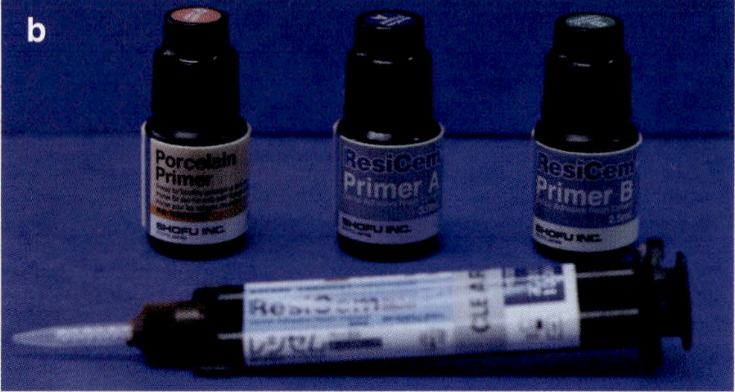

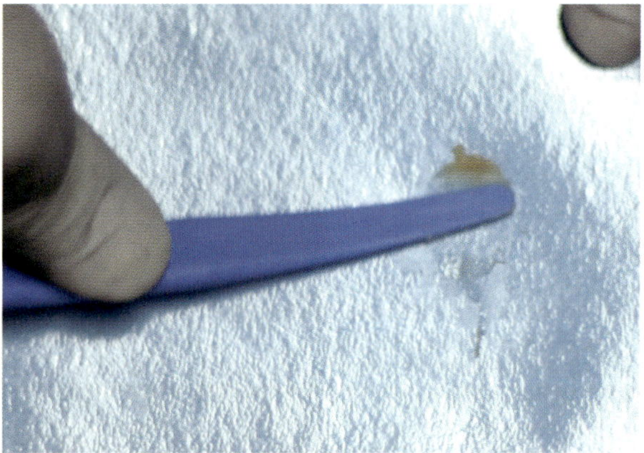

Fig. 3.9 Mixing of a two-paste resin cement using folding strokes to minimize inclusion of bubbles

a cross-linked polymer, and it also reacts chemically and micromechanically with the dentin. These cements are dual cured.

3.4.2   Clinical and Technical Considerations

The self-adhesive resin cements produce adequate bonds to the dentin and enamel. However, comparing them with etch-and-rinse and self-etch resin cements, they show lower bond strengths (Luhrs et al. 2009). Initially high bond strengths also tend to decrease with time (de Sa Barbosa et al. 2013).

As less clinical steps are needed for these cements, there is less risk of contamination, and hence these cements are not as technique sensitive as the etch-and-rinse cements. Some authors recommend their use for areas of the mouth that are difficult to isolate such as the posterior segments. Although there are reports of clinical

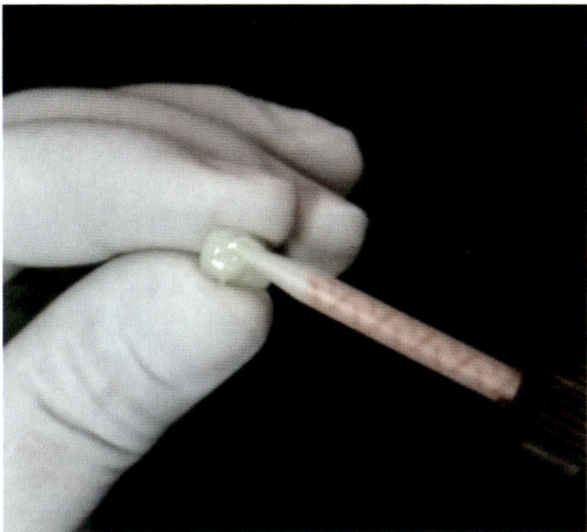

Fig. 3.10 Resin cement dispensed directly onto the restoration

success with these self-adhesive resin cements, long-term observation of their clinical success is needed as they are relatively new (Christensen 2007).

3.4.3   Indications

Self-adhesive resin cements are good alternatives to the more complicated-to-use and technique-sensitive total-etch and self-etch resin cements. They can be used for most restoration types, regardless of the restoration material except veneers. They are the resin cements of choice for high-strength ceramics such as zirconia and alumina. They are also indicated over conventional luting cements, when retention is compromised such as too tapered preparations, short crowns, and onlay preparations with little tooth structures and walls remaining and isolation and time constraints are a problem. It should be noted however that when retention is the main issue and there is a lot of dentin exposed, the self-etch resin cements should take precedence over the self-adhesive cements as self-etch cements have higher bond strengths and are more durable.

3.4.4   Manipulation

Self-adhesive resin cements come in a special double-barreled dispenser that makes it possible for the base and catalyst paste to be dispensed simultaneously and equally onto an automix tip that enables the operator to apply it directly to the restoration and preparation margins (Fig. 3.10).

As self-adhesive resin cements contain acidic monomers that degrade with heat, they should be refrigerated and kept away from sunlight.

3.5   Choice of Cement

Critical factors affecting the choice of cement are as follows:

1. Degree of retention needed which is affected by preparation design (taper of walls, length of the remaining tooth structure)
2. Ability to maintain a dry field (anterior vs. posterior teeth)
3. Aesthetics
4. Strength of the restoration material (mechanical properties)
5. Tooth bonding substrate (amount of the remaining enamel vs. amount of the remaining dentin)

Resin cements can be used for almost all types of restorations and materials, but there are situations where one type of cement is more suitable/preferable and convenient to use, yet as effective as the others. Below is a simplified guide aimed to help the clinician in choosing the most appropriate cement given a certain situation (Fig. 3.11).

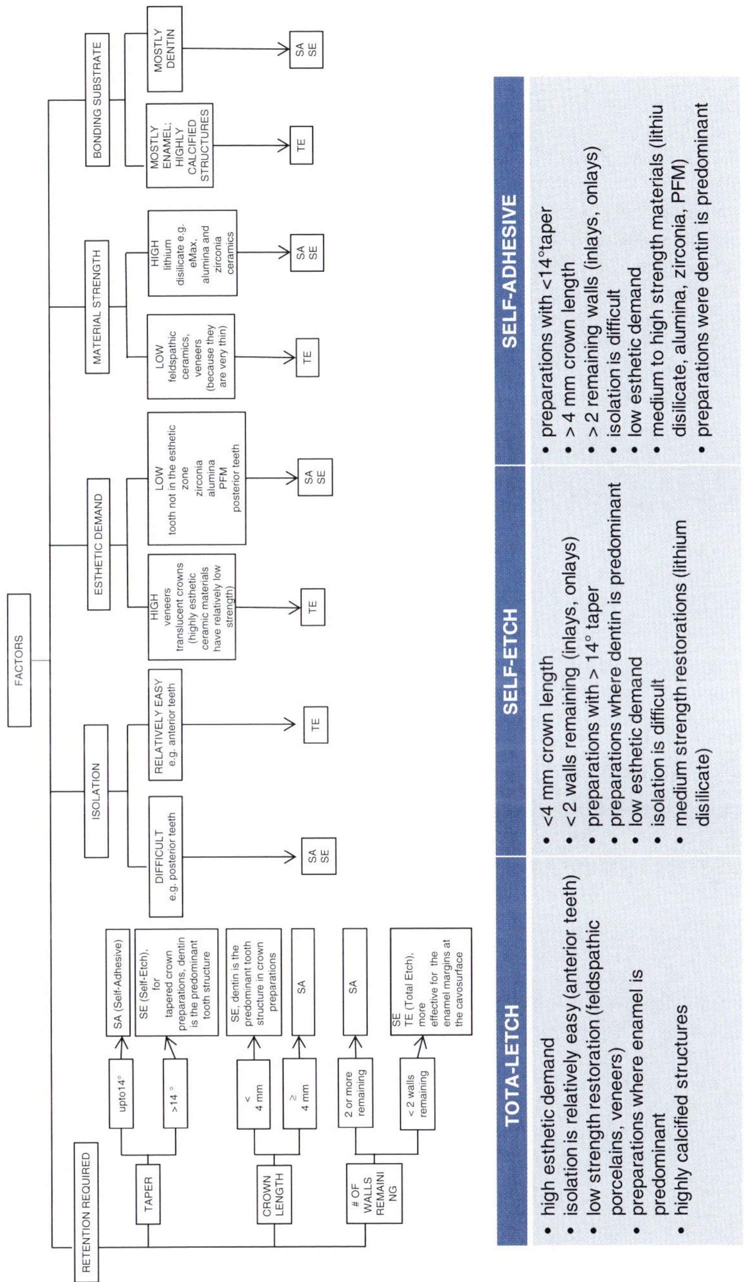

Fig. 3.11 A simplified guide to resin cement selection

References

ADA Professional Product Review (2006) Dual cure resin-based cements: expert panel discussion. Volume 1(Issue 2 (online)) www.ada.org/goto/ppr

Burgess JO, Sherman T, Cakir D (2010) Self-adhesive resin cements. J Esthet Restor Dent 22:412–417

Caselli DS, Martins LR (2006) Postoperative sensitivity in class I composite resin restorations in vivo. J Adhes Dent 8:53–58

Christensen GJ (2007) Should resin cements be used for every cementation? J Am Dent Ass 138:817–819

de Sa Barbosa NF et al (2013) Effect of water storage on bond strength of self-adhesive resin cements to zirconium oxide ceramic. J Adhes Dent 15:145–150

King NM, Tay FR, Pashley DH et al (2005) Conversion o one-step to two-step self-etch adhesives for improved efficacy and extended application. Am J Dent 18:126–134

Luhrs AK, Guhr S, Gunay H, Guertsen W et al (2009) Shear bond strength of self-adhesive resins compared to resin cements with etch and rinse adhesives to enamel and dentin in vitro. Clin Oral Investig 14:193–199

Sanvin JF, de Rijk WG (2006) Dental cements. Inside Dentistry 2:42–47

Clinical Procedures

4

4.1 Introduction

Cementation with resin cements is an adhesive procedure. The two bonding substrates, namely, the tooth surface (dentin and enamel) and the internal surface of the restoration, are usually pretreated before cementation. Cementation procedures will vary depending on the restoration material and type of resin cement. As discussed in the previous chapters, pretreatment of ceramics will differ from that of composites and metal alloys.

Being mainly adhesive, cementation with resin cements is a technique-sensitive procedure and should be done with utmost care. Each step recommended by the manufacturer has been culled from numerous researches and should be strictly followed to ensure satisfactory results. Whenever a new product is used, it is imperative that the instructions are read thoroughly before using the cement. One should remember that the composition of resin cements varies and are proprietary from brand to brand even within the same type or class of cement. One cannot assume that the instructions of one resin cement apply with another resin cement even if they are of the same type.

© Springer-Verlag Berlin Heidelberg 2015
M. Sunico-Segarra, A. Segarra, *A Practical Clinical Guide to Resin Cements*,
DOI 10.1007/978-3-662-43842-8_4

4.2   Procedural Flow Chart

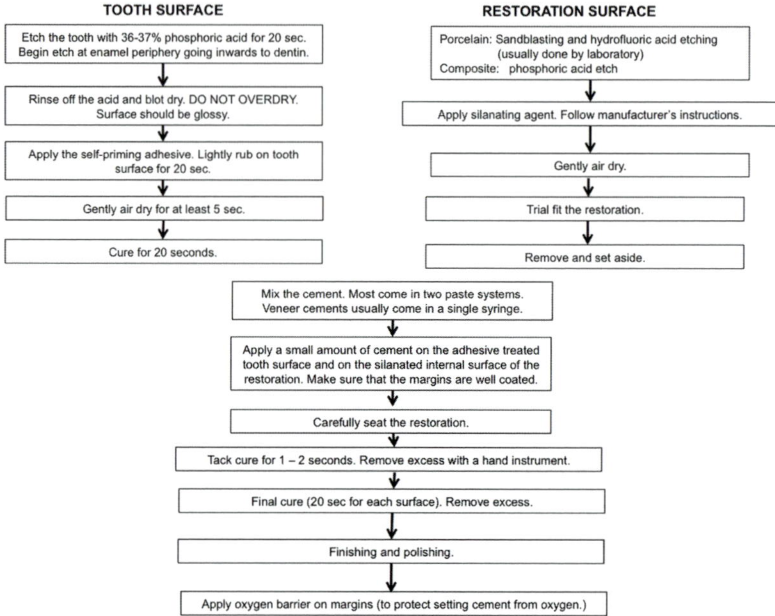

Fig. 4.1   Total-etch conventional resin cements

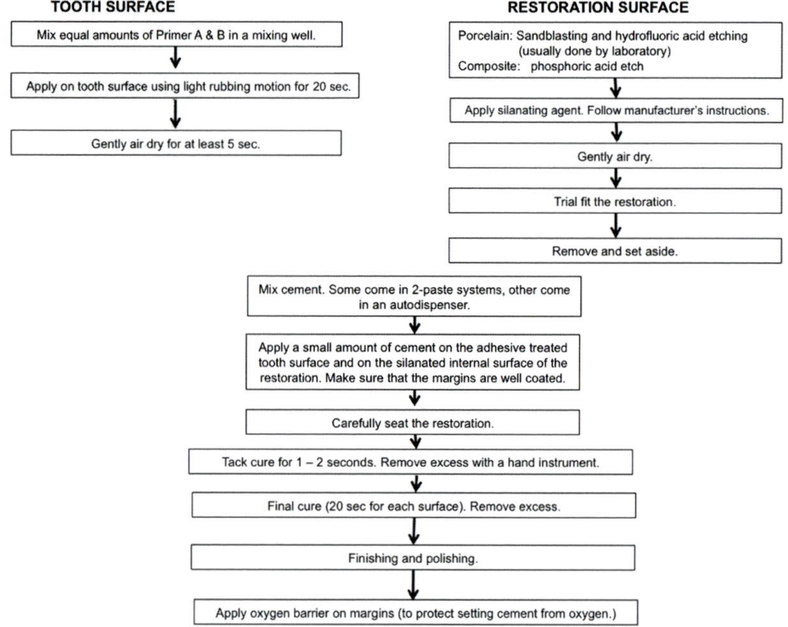

Fig. 4.2   Self-etch conventional resin cements

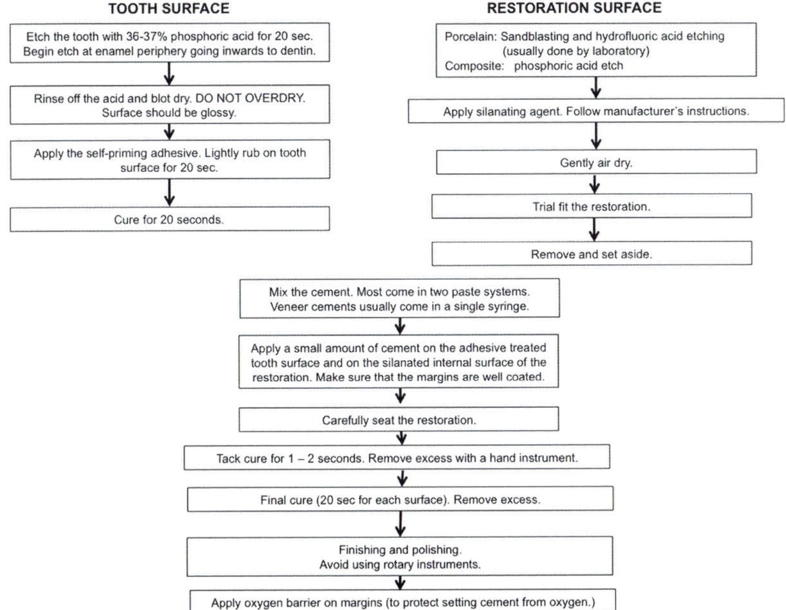

Fig. 4.3 Self-adhesive resin cements

4.3 The Resin Impregnation Technique/Immediate Dentin Seal

The use of a dentin adhesive and a low-viscosity resin to seal the dentinal tubules immediately after tooth preparation was first introduced by Nikaido et al. in 1992. This procedure was called the "resin coating or resin impregnation technique." The dentin surface of the preparation was sealed with a dentin adhesive immediately after tooth preparation followed by placement of a low-viscosity resin such as a flowable composite. This technique has been shown to reduce postoperative sensitivity during the temporization phase and increase cement bond strengths to the underlying dentin (Nikaido et al. 2003).

Magne in 2005 and Dietschi in 2002 also observed the same results with immediate sealing of the cut dentin with dentin adhesives. This procedure later became known as the "immediate dentin seal" (IDS) technique.

Several advantages have been cited for immediate dentin sealing.

Firstly, freshly cut dentin after tooth preparation is an ideal substrate for dentin bonding since contamination with provisional cements is avoided (Pashley et al. 1992).

Secondly, prepolymerization of the dentin-bonding agent results in improved bond strength. Polymerized dentin-bonding adhesive (DBA) thickness can vary significantly according to surface geometry—on average, 60–80 μm on a smooth convex surface and up to 200–300 μm on concave surfaces such as marginal chamfers. As a result, applying and polymerizing the DBA immediately before the insertion of an indirect composite resin or porcelain restoration could interfere with the complete seating of the restoration. It is therefore recommended that the adhesive resin be kept unpolymerized before the restoration is fully seated, but the pressure of the luting composite restoration can create a collapse of the demineralized dentin and affect the adhesive interface cohesiveness. It has been proposed that thinning of the adhesive layer to less than 40 μm would theoretically allow for prepolymerization before insertion of the restoration; however, because methacrylate resins show an inhibition layer of up to 40 μm thick when they are light cured (Pashley et al. 1992), excessive thinning can prevent the polymerization of light-activated dentin-bonding agents. All the aforementioned issues can be resolved if exposed dentin surfaces are sealed immediately (Magne 2005).

Thirdly, IDS allows stress-free dentin bond development. Since there is delayed placement of the restoration and postponed occlusal loading, the dentin bond can increase over time, and residual stress can dissipate resulting in improved restoration adaptation (Dietschi et al. 2002).

Finally, IDS protects dentin against bacterial leakage and sensitivity during the provisional phase of treatment which is based on research that provisional restorations may permit microleakage of bacteria and subsequently dentin sensitivity. An in vivo study confirmed the ability of different primers to prevent sensitivity and bacterial penetration when preparing for porcelain veneers (Cagidiaco et al. 1996).

4.3.1   Clinical Technique

Fig. 4.4 Inlay preparation for tooth #26

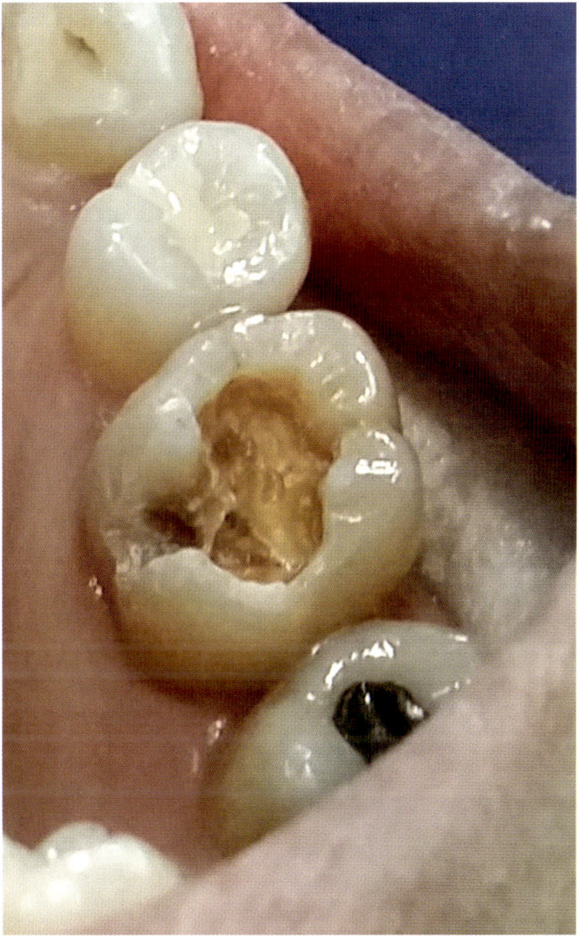

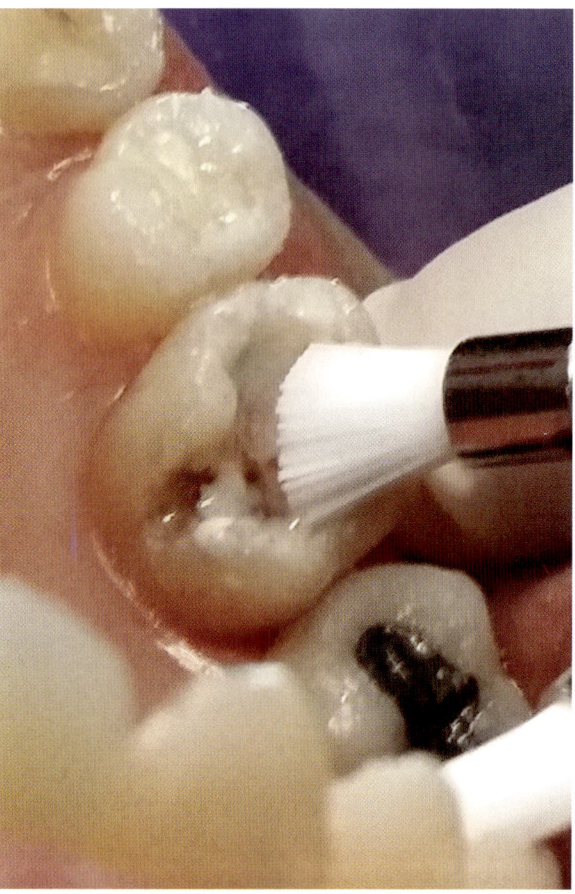

Fig. 4.5 The tooth is cleaned with a slurry of pumice to remove surface contaminants

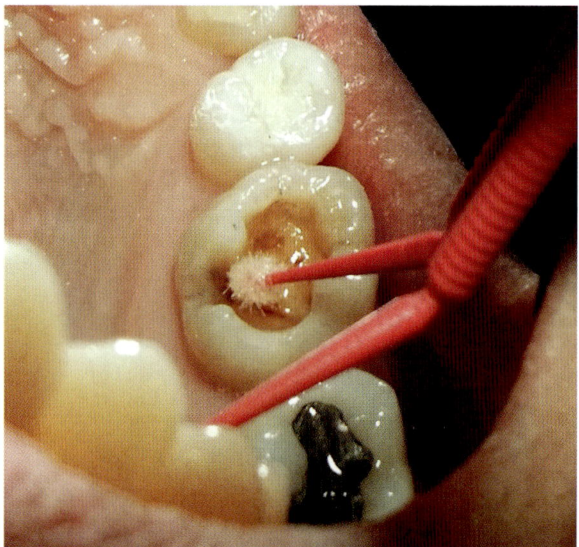

Fig. 4.6 A self-etch adhesive is used for immediate dentin sealing. The self-etch primer is applied using light rubbing motion for 20 s and then air-dried for 5–10 s

Fig. 4.7 A glossy surface after application of the self-etch primer indicating that the primer has penetrated into the dentinal tubules

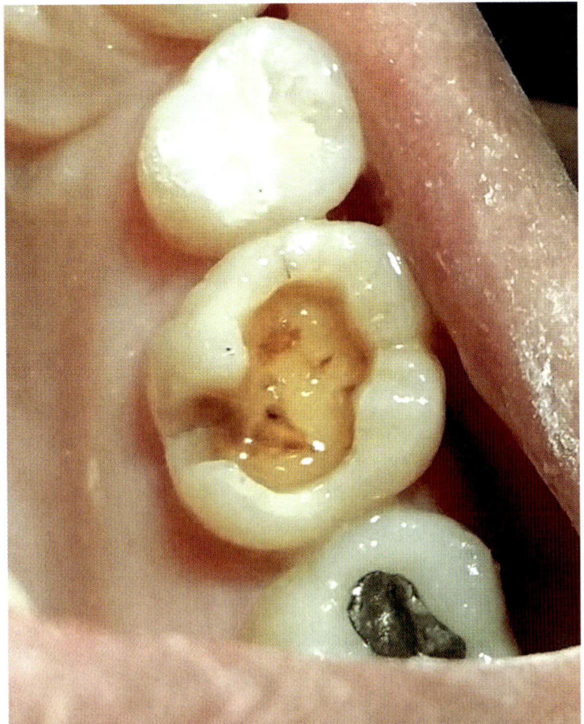

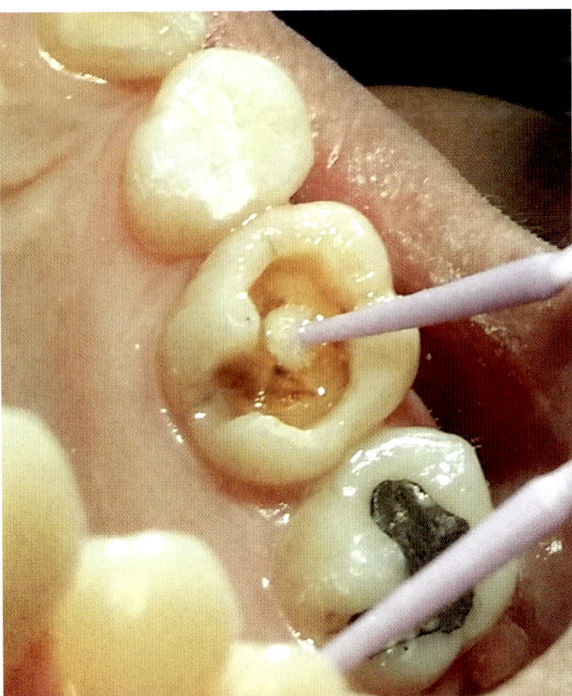

Fig. 4.8 The bonding agent is applied and air thinned

Fig. 4.9 Light curing for 10 s

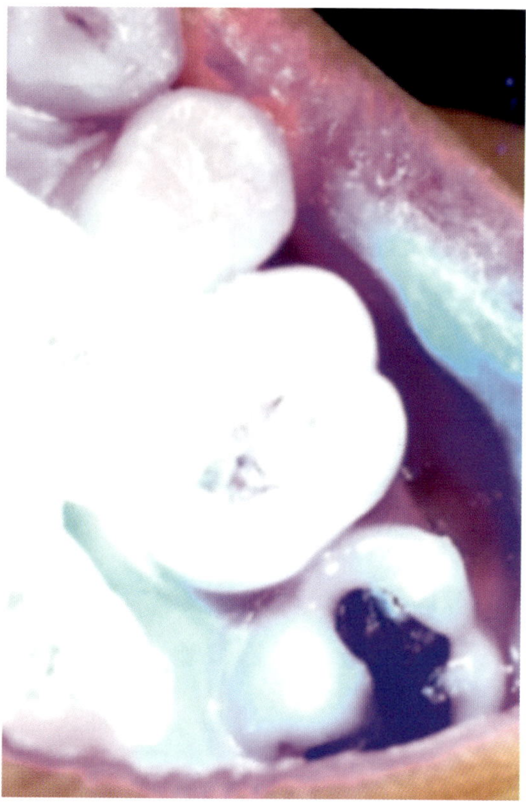

Fig. 4.10 Application of a thin layer of flowable composite or low-viscosity composite

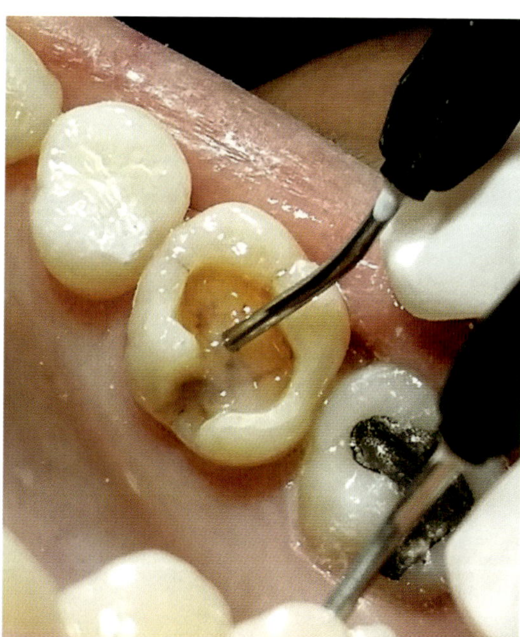

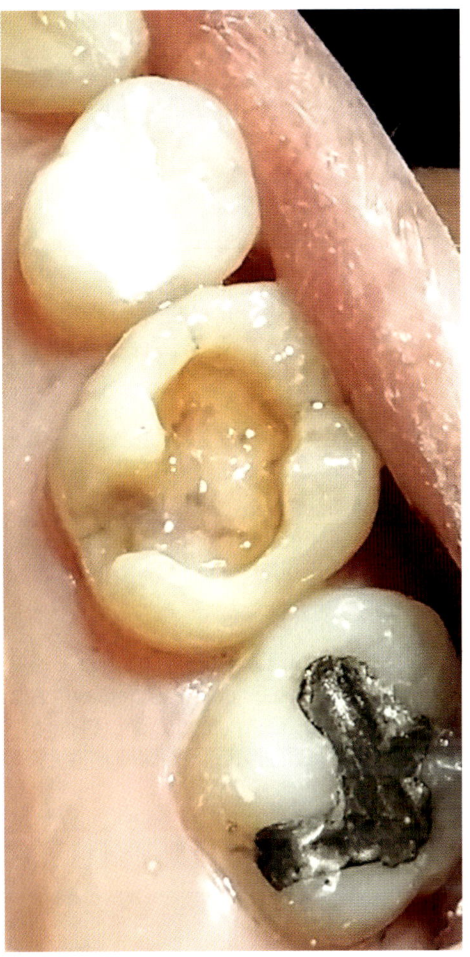

Fig. 4.11 The flowable composite is light cured. A final impression is taken

4.4 Cementation Techniques for the Different Types of Restorations

4.4.1 Tooth-Colored Inlays and Onlays

4.4.1.1 Choosing the Right Resin Cement

Preparations for inlays and onlays usually involve a lot of dentin. The inlays and onlays are usually thick (more than 2 mm). Considering these factors, the recommended cement is either a self-etch conventional resin cement or a self-adhesive resin cement. Both cements are dual cured, and thus, they will cure underneath a thick restoration. The choice between the self-etch conventional or self-adhesive resin cement will depend on the degree of retention needed. For preparations with few remaining walls (Fig. 4.12), the self-etch resin cement, when available, can be chosen over the self-adhesive resin cement.

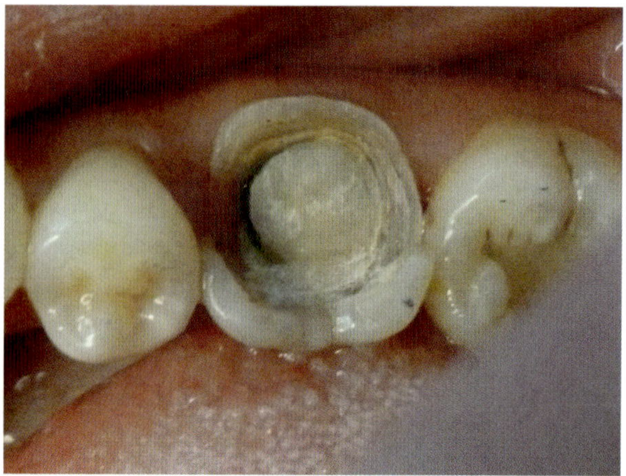

Fig. 4.12 Onlay preparation with very few remaining walls. Retention is compromised. Although both a conventional self-etch resin cement and a self-adhesive resin cement can be used, a conventional self-etch resin cement is a better choice

A flowable composite should never be used to cement thick tooth-colored inlays and onlays as light will not penetrate through the thick material resulting to inadequate polymerization. This may cause pulpal death from the unreacted monomers.

4.4.1.2 Clinical Case

Laboratory fabricated composite inlays (Adoro) on teeth # 26 and 27 to be cemented with a self-adhesive resin cement (Clearfil SA Luting, Kuraray, Japan). The inlays were sandblasted by the laboratory.

Fig. 4.13 The tooth was cleaned with a slurry of pumice to remove surface debris that may interfere with bonding

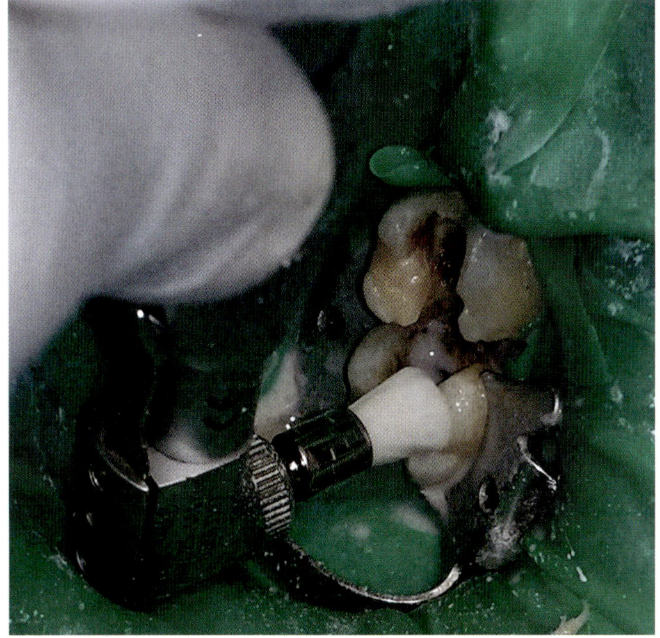

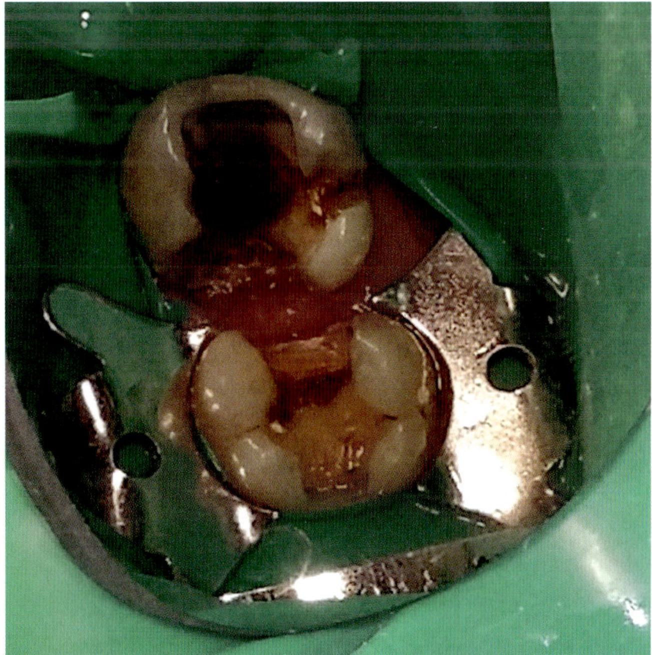

Fig. 4.14 The prepared teeth. To ensure good bonding, obtain proper isolation

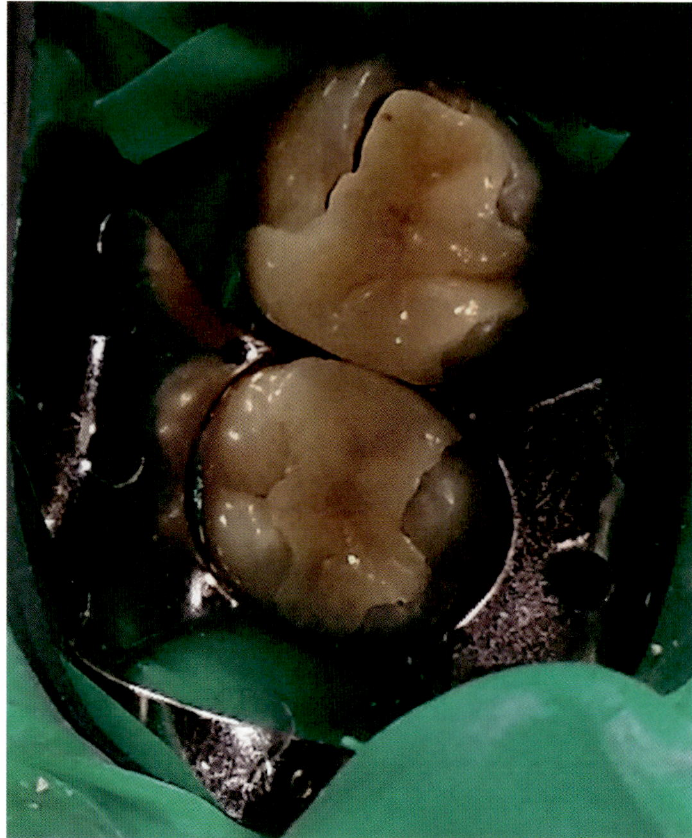

Fig. 4.15 Trial fitting of the inlays. Notice a slight gap on the mesiobuccal area of 26 indicating the inlay has not seated properly. This might have been caused by a prematurity, irregularity, or bubbles on the internal surface of the restoration or a prematurity on the proximal contacts of 26 and 27. The prematurities were identified with a fit checker and articulating paper and subsequently trimmed

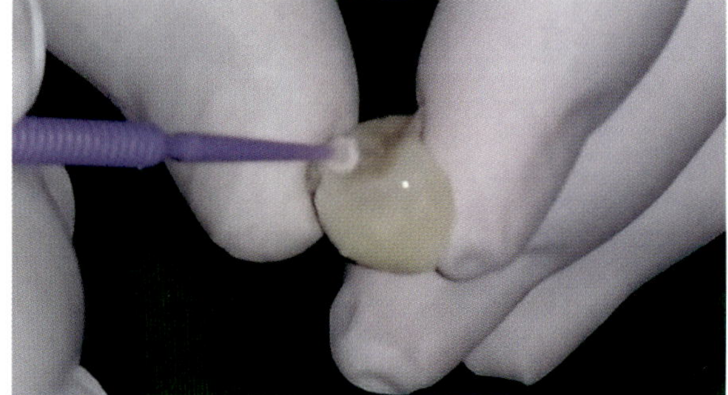

Fig. 4.16 The external surface of the inlay was coated with a thin layer of petroleum jelly to facilitate subsequent clean up. Care was taken not to inadvertently place petroleum jelly on the adhesive surfaces

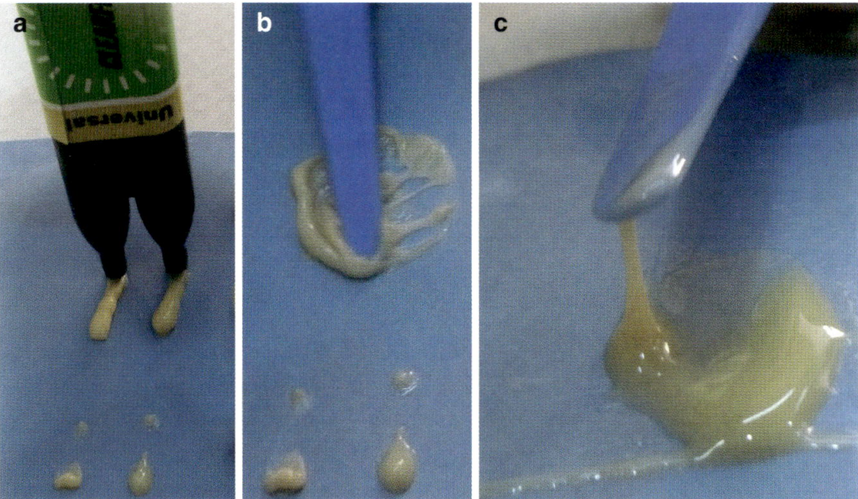

Fig. 4.17 (**a**) A self-adhesive resin cement (Clearfil SA Luting, Kuraray, Japan) is dispensed on a mixing pad. (**b**) The two pastes are mixed thoroughly using folding strokes to prevent incorporation of air. (**c**) Properly mixed cement. The cement should string 2 cm from the mixing pad

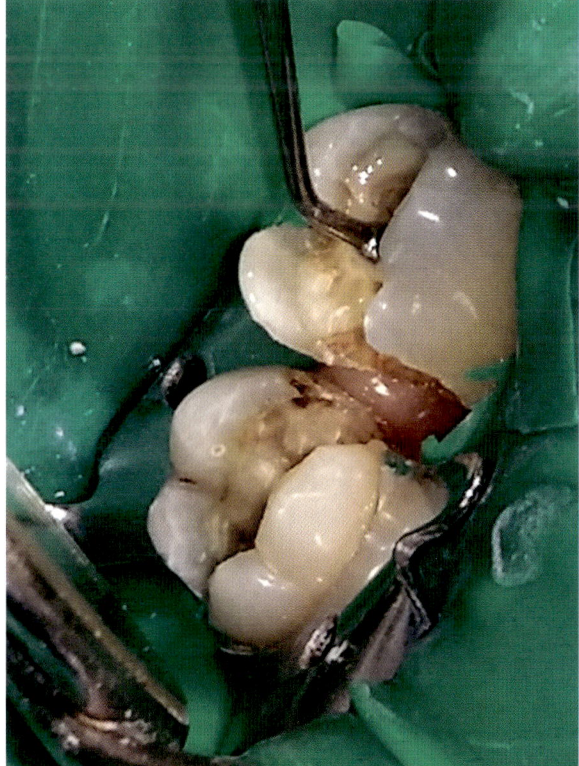

Fig. 4.18 A small amount of resin cement was wiped into the cavity preparation to ensure that the internal walls are well coated with cement and to minimize voids

Fig. 4.19 To ensure that the critical gingival margin is sealed, a small amount of resin cement is also wiped onto the gingival floor and proximal margins

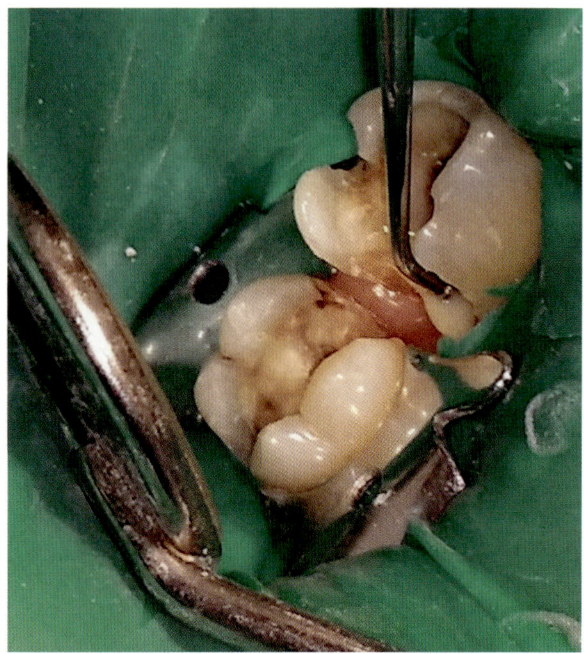

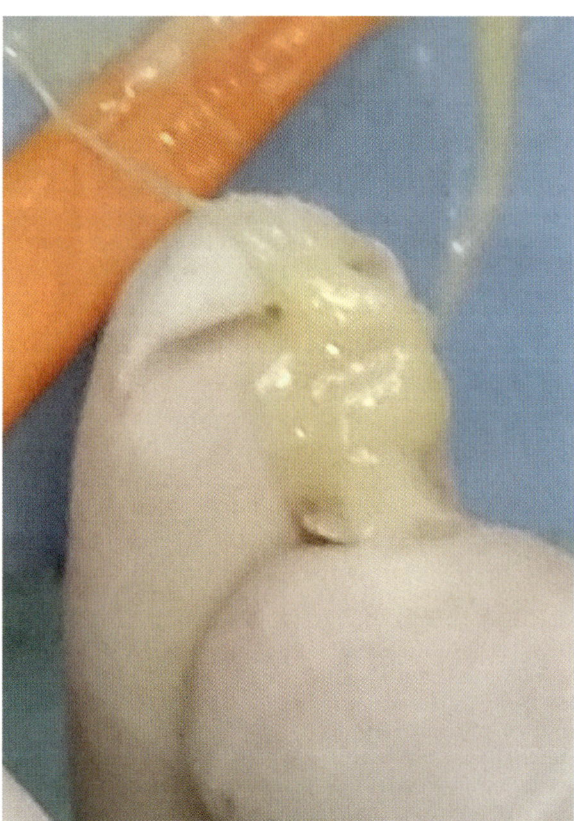

Fig. 4.20 The internal surface of the restoration was also coated with resin cement

Fig. 4.21 The 26 onlay was then seated on the prepared tooth using slow, gentle pressure. Do not seat the restoration using strong abrupt force as this may create pressure to build up between the walls of the tooth and the restoration which might push the restoration occlusally. A slow steady pressure will give enough time for the excess cement to flow out aiding in the proper seating of the restoration

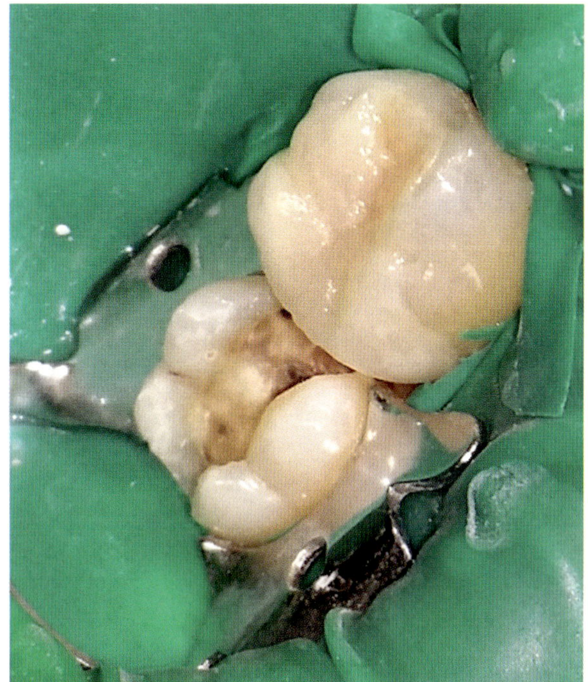

Fig. 4.22 The cement was cured for 1–2 s (tack curing or tack and wave technique). The cement is not cured completely until all excess cement is removed. Tack curing renders the cement partially set and gives the excess cement a consistency that is easy to peel off from the tooth and restoration for a very easy clean up

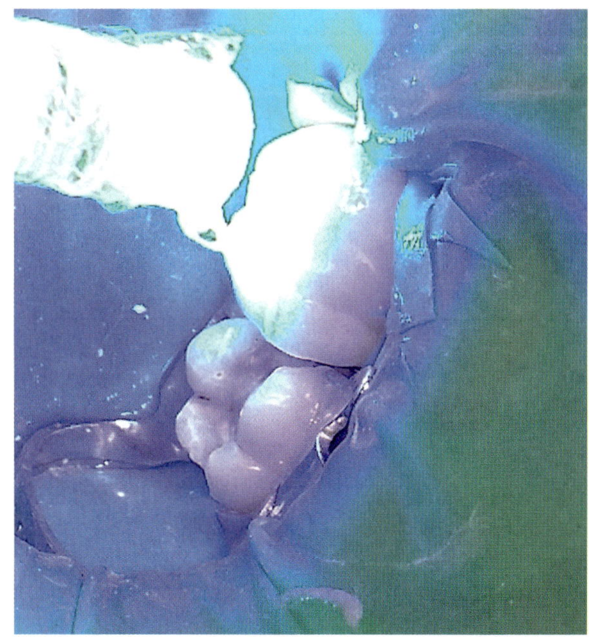

Fig. 4.23 Excess cement was carefully removed from the surface of the restoration. Note the consistency of the tack-cured cement. Care should be taken not to remove any cement between the restoration and the cavosurface margin. When there is a slight gap between restoration and the tooth, a clean brush is used to remove excess cement prior to curing, to protect the fragile "cement seal" between the tooth and restoration. Tack curing when there is a slight gap may just pull out the cement from the interface

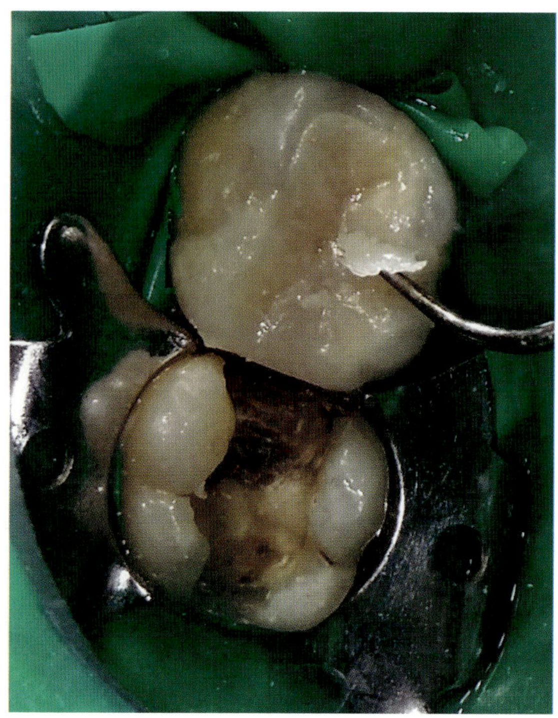

Fig. 4.24 The second inlay is fitted. An articulating paper inserted between the two inlays is used to check for any prematurities in the proximal area

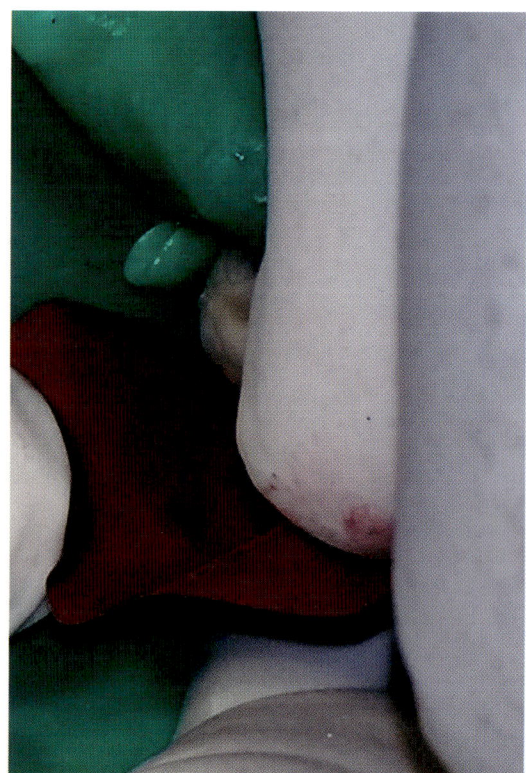

Fig. 4.25 Note the mark made by the articulating paper. The marked area is a prematurity that prevents complete seating of the inlay. The inlay is then trimmed (on the die) removing the prematurity. Never trim the inlay without the die to avoid fracture

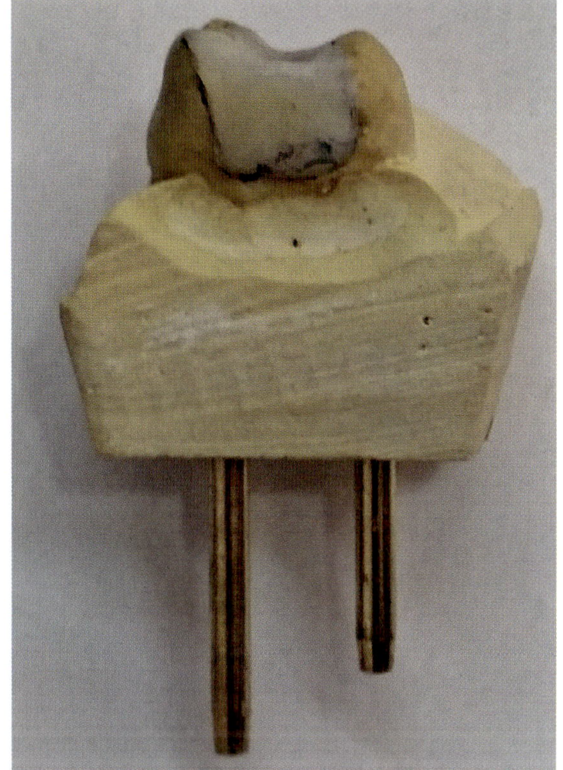

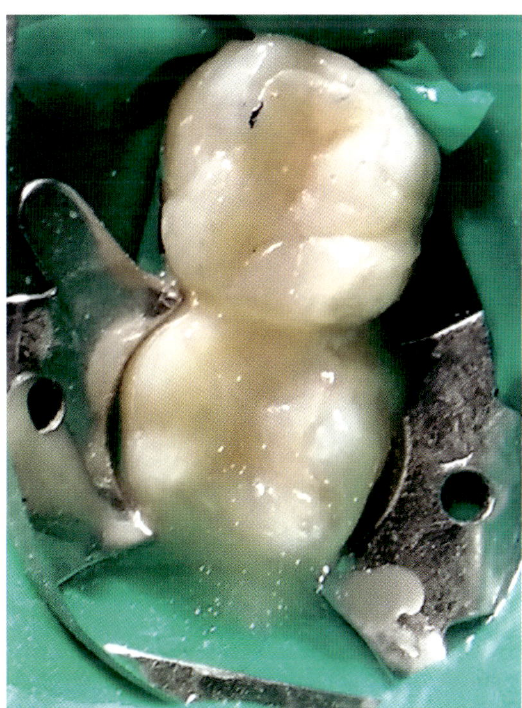

Fig. 4.26 The second inlay (27) was seated and cemented using the same cementation technique

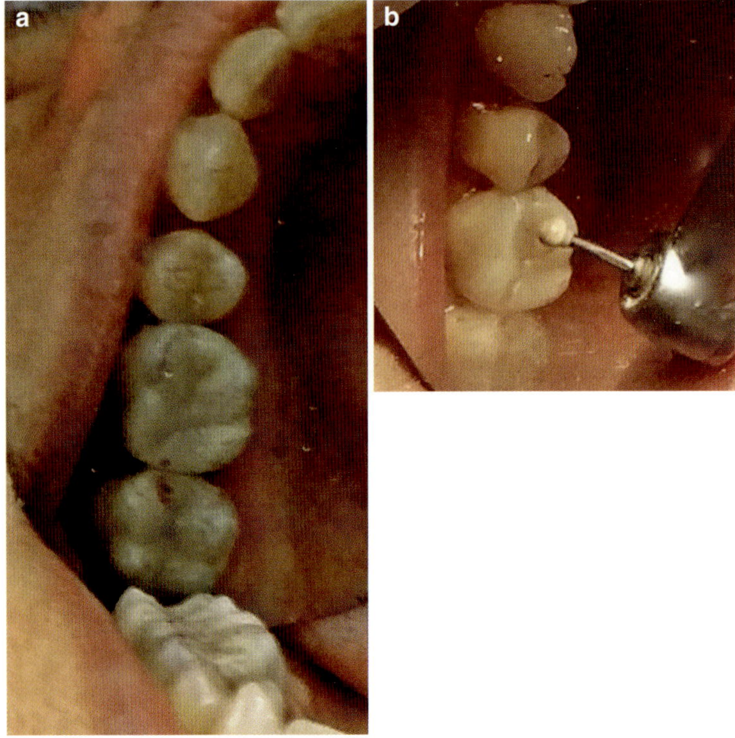

Fig. 4.27 Occlusal adjustment. Occlusal adjustment is done only after the onlay is cemented. (**a**) The patient was asked to bite on an articulating paper to identify occlusal prematurities (high spots). (**b**) The prematurities were removed with a composite trimmer

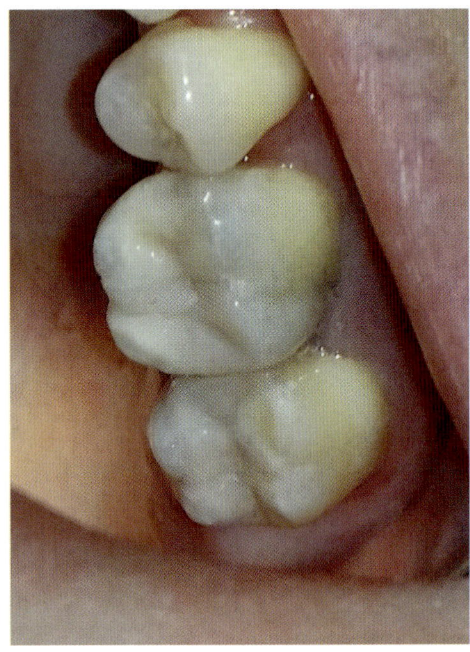

Fig. 4.28 The cemented inlays

4.4.1.3 Trial Fitting an Inlay/Onlay

One of the difficulties during the cementation procedure is placing the inlay on the preparation. Inlays/onlays are very small and fragile, and there is also the danger of the patient swallowing these restorations. Rubber dam isolation is always a good practice during trial fitting and cementation of inlays.

Several techniques have been suggested in the dental literature:

1. Use of a "sticky stick" to hold the restoration during fitting. The stick will serve as a "handle" for the inlay. These sticks are commercially available or can be improvised.

McLaren and Hamilton suggest two techniques for improvising an inlay or veneer "handle." The surface of the inlay is first wiped with isopropyl alcohol. A microbrush or adhesive applicator is dipped into a bonding agent (not the primer-adhesive combinations, but the bonding agent of two-step self-etch systems as they are not acidic) and light cured onto the inlay. After cementation, the handle can be easily removed with a curette.

The other technique is to use a sticky wax instead of a bonding agent. The sticky wax is heated either with a Bunsen burner, electronic waxer, or alcohol torch and attached onto the surface of the inlay. To remove the handle after cementation, the wax is sprayed with water and the handle is flicked off.

2. Use of a Teflon tape or "dental white tape."

Geissberger et al. (2002) described a procedure where Teflon tape is used as a "liner" for fitting inlays. A thin layer of Teflon tape is lined inside the cavity preparation prior to seating of the inlay. This method facilitates removal of the inlay after try-in. A knot is tied close to the occlusal surface of the restoration prior to its removal to protect against inadvertent loss or swallowing. After assessing the fit, the Teflon tape can be easily removed together with the inlay.

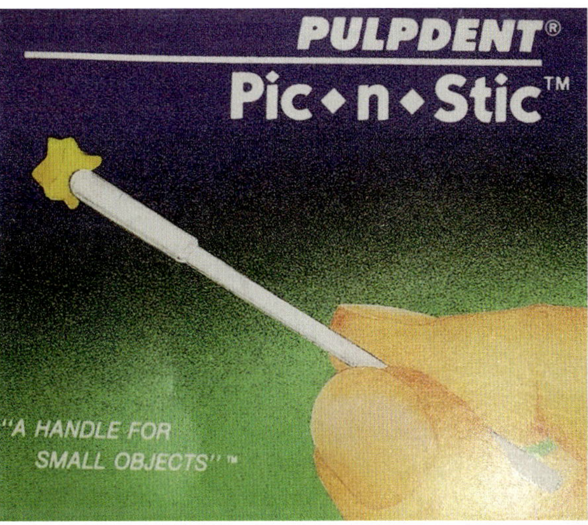

Fig. 4.29 Pic-n-Stic (Pulpdent, USA)

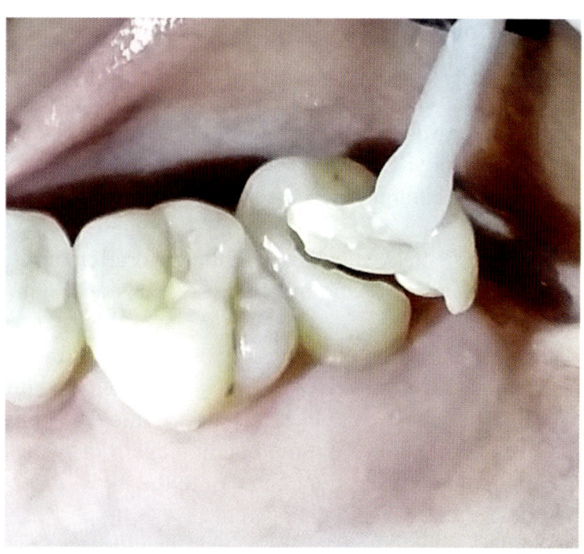

Fig. 4.30 Pic-n-Stic used to position an onlay on tooth #27

4.4.1.4 Points to Remember

1. Use a dual-cured cement for onlays/inlays. Flowable composites are *not* for cementation of inlays/onlays as the light cannot penetrate through the thick restorations.
2. Follow manufacturer's instructions. For best results, equal amounts of the base and catalyst paste should be dispensed and thoroughly mixed. It is not possible to use only one paste as the composition of Paste A and Paste B are different and are both needed to ensure good bonding and clinical results. This is especially true for the self-etch conventional resin cements and self-adhesive resin cements which usually come in double-barreled syringes.
3. As cementation with resin cements is an adhesive procedure, isolation is a necessity to prevent contamination, which may compromise bonding.
4. Dual-cured cements need to be light cured.
5. Adjust the occlusion only after the inlay is cemented to avoid inadvertent loss or fracture of the restoration.
6. Make sure that all gross cement excess is removed prior to final curing as completely cured cement is difficult to clean up.

4.4.2 Porcelain Veneer Restorations

4.4.2.1 Choosing the Right Cement

The retention of veneers depends mainly on the cementing medium. Unlike other indirect restorations such as crowns and inlays where there are several walls to retain them, veneers lack the necessary retention and resistance form as it is usually bonded only to the labial surface.

Another important consideration in selecting veneer cement is esthetics. As veneers are oftentimes very thin restorations, the cementing material should exhibit high color stability as any discoloration can show through the very thin veneer and affect overall esthetics. Selection of the proper cement is thus very critical to the success of the restoration.

1. Choose an etch-and-rinse resin cement, also called *total-etch resin cements.*
As veneer preparations should ideally be limited on the enamel, aggressive etching with phosphoric acid is preferable over milder etching obtained with self-etch systems.

2. A resin cement that polymerizes exclusively by *light curing.*
The thinness of veneers requires very color stable cement. Dual-cured resin cements contain amine co-initiators which tend to discolor and turn yellow over time, one reason why they are not recommended for cementation of veneers less than 0.5 mm thick.
Light-cured resin cements are more color stable as the initiator used is camphoroquinone. However, the cement should be light polymerized completely as unreacted camphoroquinone will also undergo yellowing over time. Thus, they are the cement of choice for thin veneers. Light-activated cements usually come as a single syringe and require no mixing. They are dispensed directly from the syringe.
Color shift becomes not much of a factor with thicker veneers, such as those used to correct teeth that are lingually positioned. A dual-cured resin cement might even be more preferable than light-cured cements as the light may not be able to polymerize the cement through the thick veneer.

4.4.2.2 Examples of Veneer Cements

Examples of resin cements specifically recommended for cementation of veneers include RelyX Veneer (3 M Espe), Choice 2 (Bisco), NX3 Veneer Cement (Kerr), Calibra (Dentsply Caulk), Variolink Veneer Cement (Vivadent), and Mojo Veneer Cement (Pentron). Calibra is a universal cement system, and it can be used for all types of tooth-colored indirect restorations. When used to cement veneers, only the base paste is used and it becomes completely light activated.

4.4.2.3 Flowable Composites to Cement Veneers

There is conflicting evidence on the viability of flowable composites as cement for veneers. A study in 2003 by Barceleiro et al. showed that flowable composites can be used as an alternative to resin veneer cements in terms of bond strength. However, a similar study by Esmaili et al. in 2007 yielded a different result and showed that flowable composites are inferior to resin veneer cements in terms of bond strength. As they also polymerize exclusively by light activation and can be used in conjunction with total-etch adhesives, it is expected that some clinicians would use it for veneer cementation in lieu of the veneer cements. Flowable composites, however, cannot be used to cement veneers that are more than 1 mm thick as light might not be able to penetrate through the veneer and cause inadequate polymerization of the composite. Care should be taken that the flowable composite attains the same film thickness (25 μm) and flow characteristics of a veneer cement. A too thick film thickness can induce stresses during seating and may cause fracture of the thin veneer. A suggested method to improve flow characteristics is to warm the composite in hot water or in an electric warmer prior to cementation.

Another consideration when using flowable composites to cement veneers is the filler loading of the flowable composite. The flowable composite should have a high filler content (71–84 % filler by weight) to ensure maximum strength.

4.4.2.4 Selecting the Resin Cement Shade

Generally, the shade of the cement should match the shade of the veneer. Translucent cements will give a more natural appearance and is considered a "safe" shade for teeth with no discolorations. Opaque cements are used to block the darkness of severely discolored teeth. However, for teeth with severe discolorations, the use of very opaque cements may give an unnatural appearance. Use of dentin modifiers on the tooth might be a better option (Munoz-Viveros, accessed 2012).

4.4.2.5 Try-In Pastes

Try-in pastes give a pretty good estimate on the final shade of the veneer after final cementation. However, differences have been found between try-in pastes and the cured resin cement of the same shade (Munoz-Viveros, accessed 2012). Try-in pastes should also be completely water soluble to ensure easy cleanup.

Try-in pastes can be useful in verifying the final shade and allows the clinician to make minor shade modifications. A technique suggested by McLaren and Hamilton in 2007 is to start with a clear try-in paste to see if the bonded veneer has the desired value (degree of brightness or darkness). If the veneer lacks brightness, they recommend adding opaque to the clear try-in paste in 5 % increments until the desired value is obtained. However, opacity of more than 25 % can give the veneer an unnaturally white appearance.

4.4.2.6 Cementation of Multiple Veneers

The sequence of seating multiple veneers will differ from one clinician to another. Some prefer to cement them all at once, some cement their veneers one at a time, and some prefer to cement them two at a time starting with the centrals and moving posteriorly in pairs. Although seating and cementing multiple veneers all at once may be fast, cement cleanup might be very difficult. Another problem is that the cement might splint the teeth together making cleanup more difficult.

Cementing veneers one at a time may give better control of the procedure, easier cleanup, and better overall esthetics as adjustments on the proximals can be done equally on both sides should there be overcrowding of the veneers. The adjacent teeth can also be isolated to prevent accidental "splinting" by stretching a very thin piece of Teflon tape material or "plumbers" tape over the contact area of the adjacent tooth, a procedure first described by Liebenberg. The tape protects the adjacent tooth from accidental etching, bonding, and eventual splinting.

4.4.2.7 The "Tack and Wave" Technique

The tack and wave technique introduced by Dr. David Hornbrook (Hornbrook Accessed 2012) is one method of light curing cements under veneer restorations. In this technique, the restorations are seated on the teeth and cured for 1 s on the center with a small-diameter light guide. The restoration is cured again, this time with a larger diameter light guide waved about one inch from the restorations for an additional 3 s, allowing the cement to establish a "semi-gel state." This technique of curing cements enables the veneers to be initially seated without them drifting or falling off. Another benefit of this technique is that the cement achieves enough body for the excess to be easily peeled off from the gingival and interproximal margins before final polymerization.

4.4.2.8 Cement Cleanup

Once the restoration is seated, excess cement should be removed with a clean brush and then cured into place using the "tack and wave" technique. After peeling off excess cement from the gingival and interproximal margins, the cement is polymerized completely, about 20 s. Any remaining excess cement can be removed with a curette or a #12 blade on a Bard-Parker scalpel handle. Avoid using rotary instruments especially on the gingival area/margins as the porcelain in this area is thin and can fracture. Also, the original gloss and polish should be retained for gingival health.

A post-installation appointment should be scheduled a few days after the final cementation to check if there is still excess cement left.

4.4.2.9 Cementation of Subgingival Veneers

A common problem during cementation of subgingival veneers is contamination from gingival bleeding or from the sulcular fluid. The gingival tissue may unseat the veneer, excess cement may seep into the sulcus, and sulcular fluid or blood can seep between the veneer and the tooth causing contamination. This compromises the bond on the very critical gingival margins and can also cause discoloration.

A good method of cementing subgingival veneers is to seat it only 90 % of the way, clean excess cement with a brush, and then seat completely. Tack cure, remove excess cement with a periodontal curette or scaler, and then cure completely.

Whether the veneer is supra- or subgingival, it is a good practice to place a retraction cord prior to final fitting and cementation.

4.4.2.10 Storage and Handling of Veneer Cements

Veneer cements can be stored at room temperature. It is not necessary to refrigerate them as cooling can affect their flow characteristics (Chadwick et al. 2008). If they are refrigerated, they should be allowed to revert to room temperature or even warmer prior to use (Munoz-Viveros, accessed 2012).

4.4.2.11 Clinical Case

Porcelain veneer restorations on maxillary anterior teeth

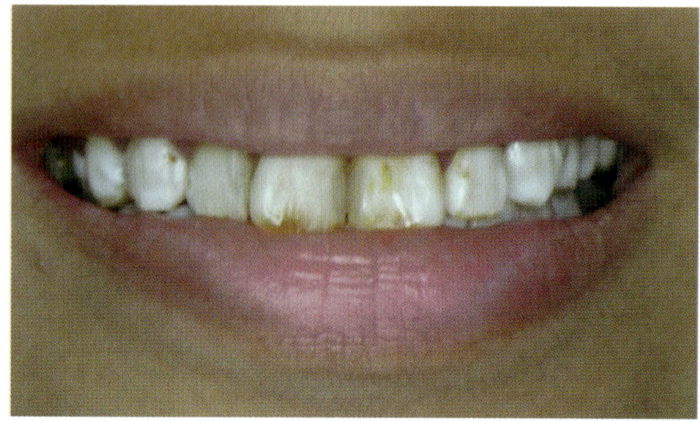

Fig. 4.31 A mild case of dental fluorosis. Porcelain veneers will be placed on the sixth maxillary anterior teeth

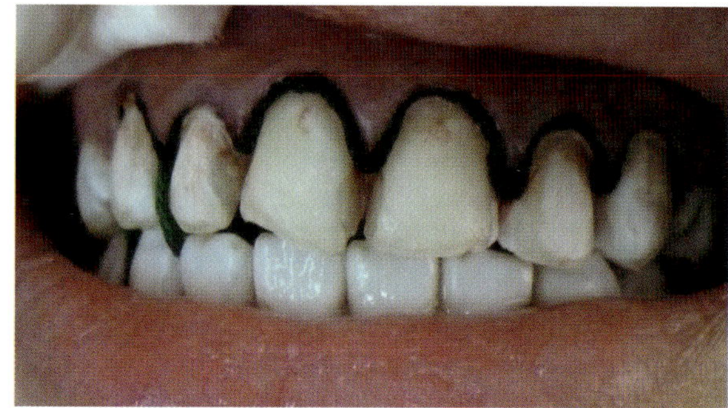

Fig. 4.32 The veneer preparations, retraction cords in place. Note that the preparations remain on the enamel avoiding exposure of the dentin

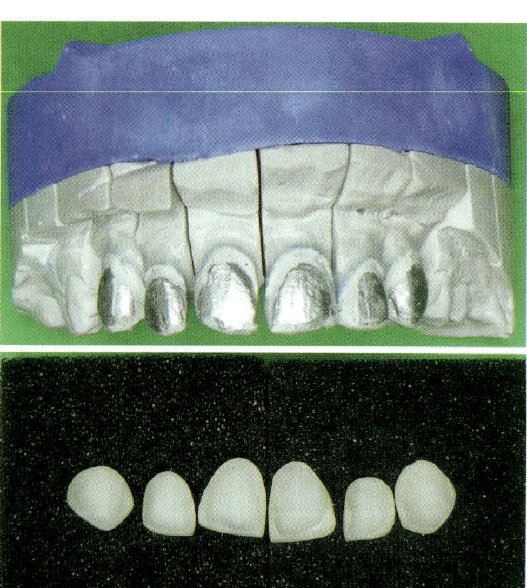

Fig. 4.33 The six porcelain veneers

Fig. 4.34 (**a**) If the veneers were not etched or sandblasted by the laboratory, the tissue surface of the veneers are etched with hydrofluoric acid (HFA). (**b**) An example of a porcelain etchant containing 9 % hydrofluoric acid (porcelain etchant, Pulpdent USA). Hydrofluoric acid should be handled with care as it may cause burns

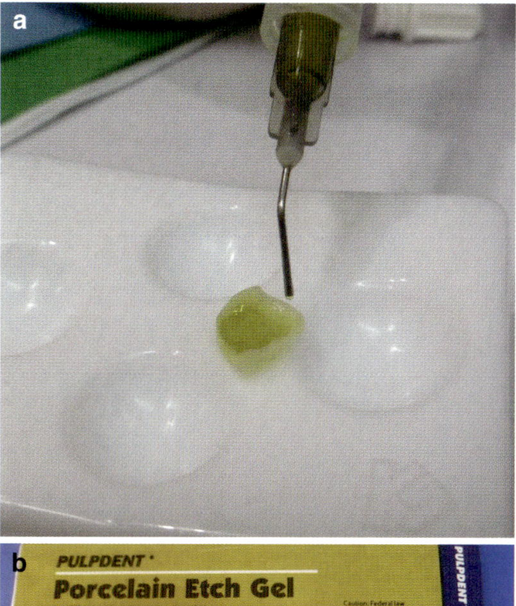

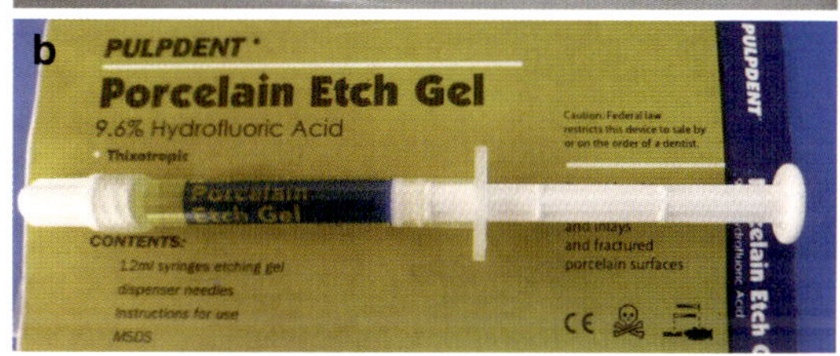

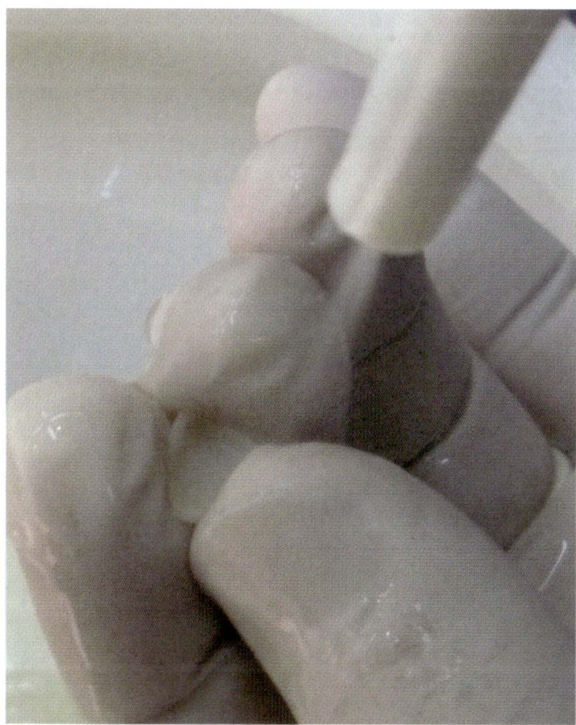

Fig. 4.35 The porcelain etchant is washed off with copious amount of water, and the veneers are dried

Fig. 4.36 (**a**) Silane was applied on the internal surfaces of the porcelain veneers and left for 1 and a half minutes, as per manufacturer's instructions. (**b**) An example of a silane (Pulpdent, USA)

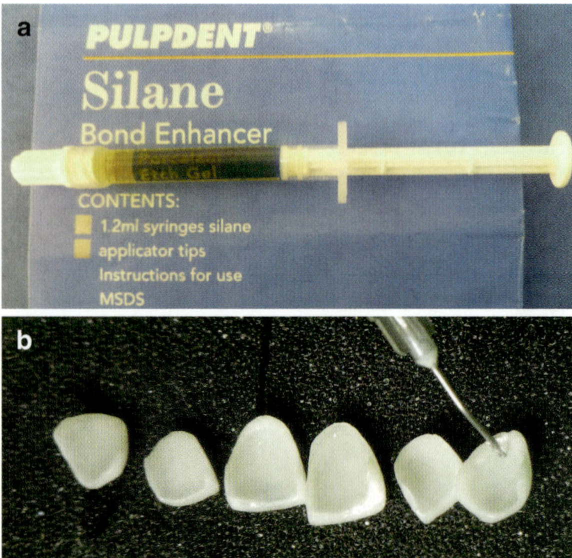

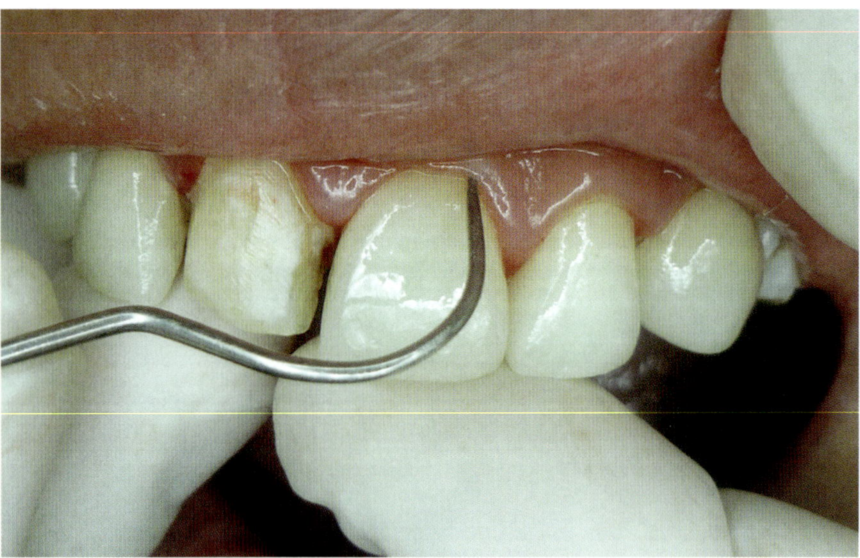

Fig. 4.37 Trial fitting of the veneers. Each veneer was fitted and checked for fit especially on the margins. A "handle" (see Sect. 4.4, page 57, Fig. 4.29) can be used to facilitate try-in of the veneers

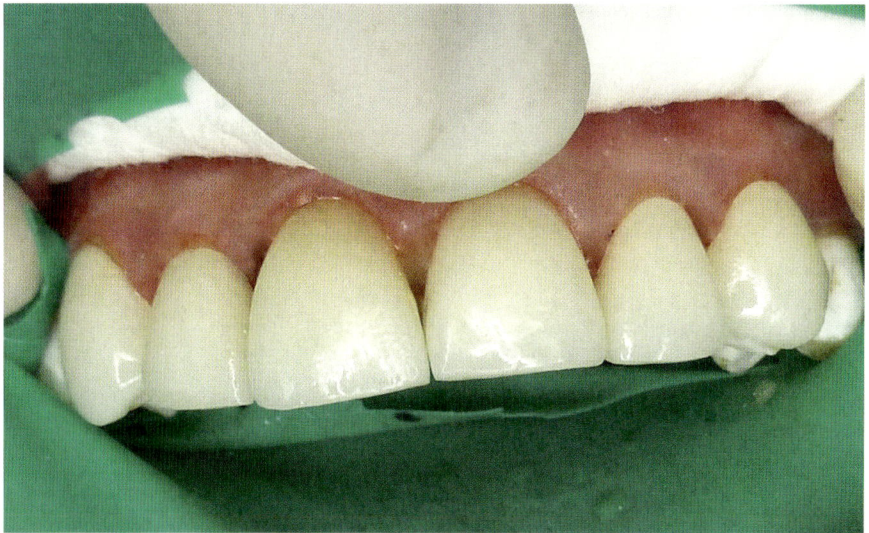

Fig. 4.38 The six veneers seated and checked for fit and esthetics

Fig. 4.39 The prepared teeth etched with 36 % phosphoric acid for 20 s. The etchant was thoroughly rinsed with water for 60 s

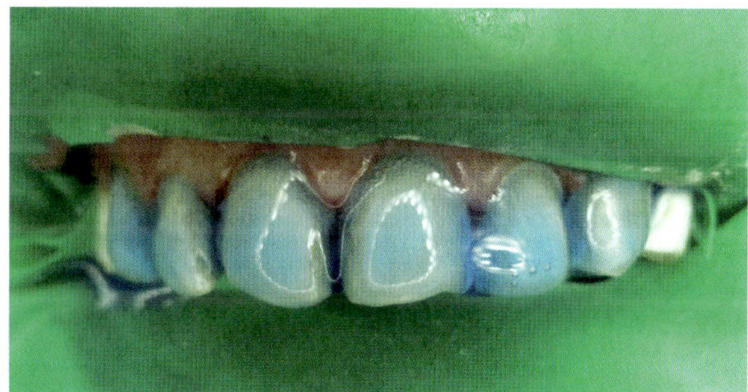

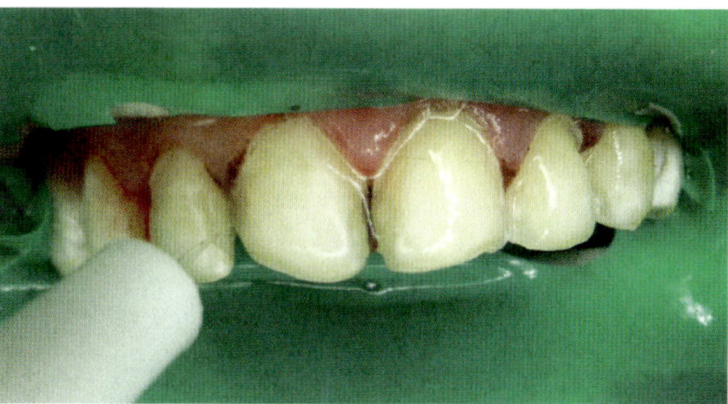

Fig. 4.40 The teeth were lightly air-dried

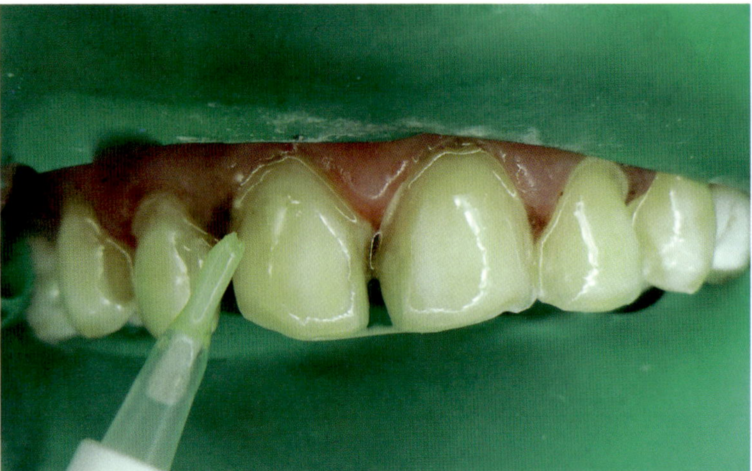

Fig. 4.41 The self-priming adhesive applied on the etched teeth for 20 s

Fig. 4.42 The adhesive is air-dried to remove excess solvent and moisture which may interfere with bonding

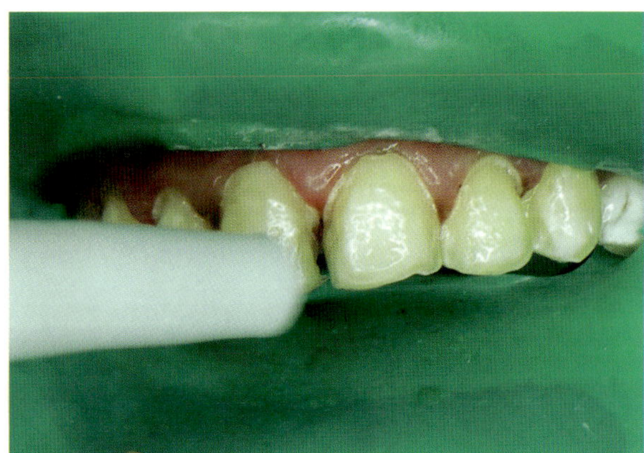

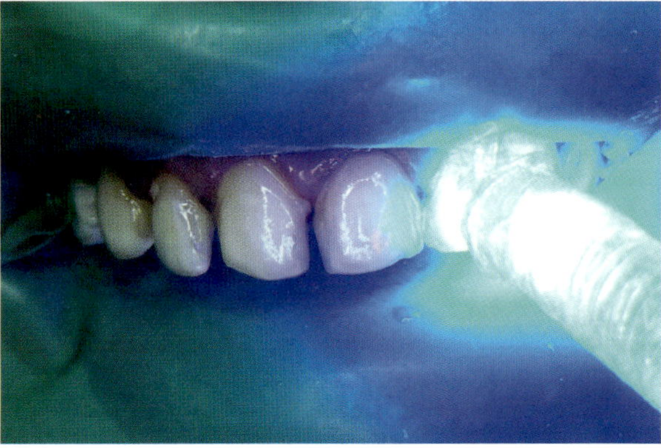

Fig. 4.43 Twenty seconds light curing for each tooth

Fig. 4.44 The Nexus 3 cement kit (Kerr, USA). The double-barreled cements on the left are the self-adhesive resin cements. They come in base-catalyst pastes. The single-syringe cements are the veneer cements, and there is no catalyst paste. Polymerization is completely by light curing

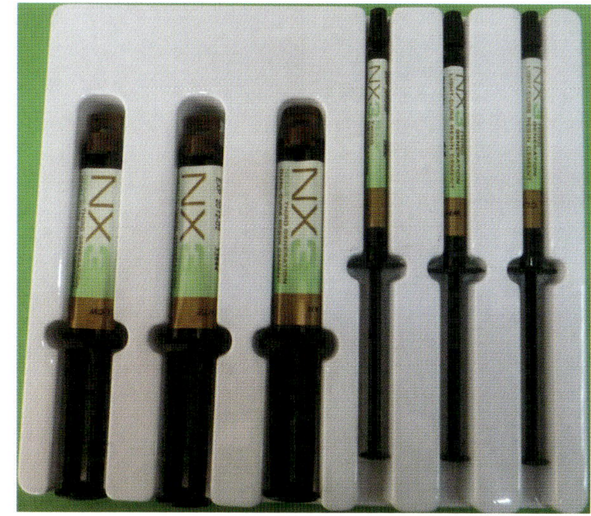

Fig. 4.45 The veneer cement loaded on the porcelain veneer

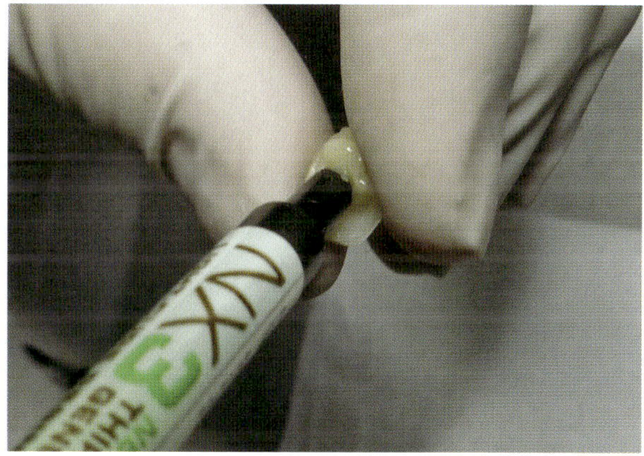

Fig. 4.46 The veneers are seated. Excess cement was initially removed with a clean brush so as not to remove the fragile cement line on the gingival margins

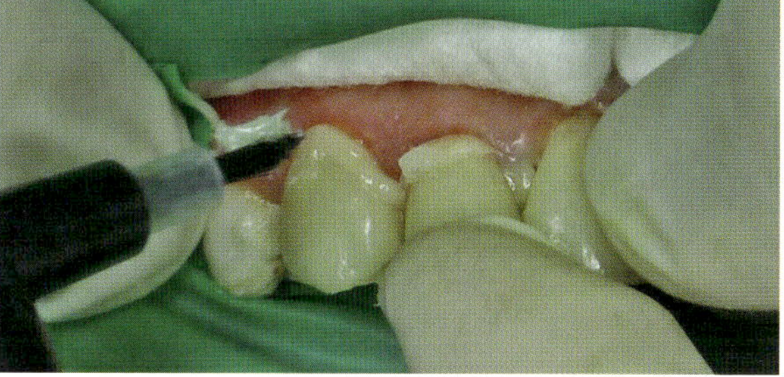

Fig. 4.47 Once the veneers are properly positioned and excess cement is initially removed with a clean brush, the veneers are tack cured in the middle of the labial surface one veneer at a time. The tack curing is to stabilize the veneers, while the alignment and position of the veneers are checked for the final time. This way, minor adjustments can still be made prior to final curing

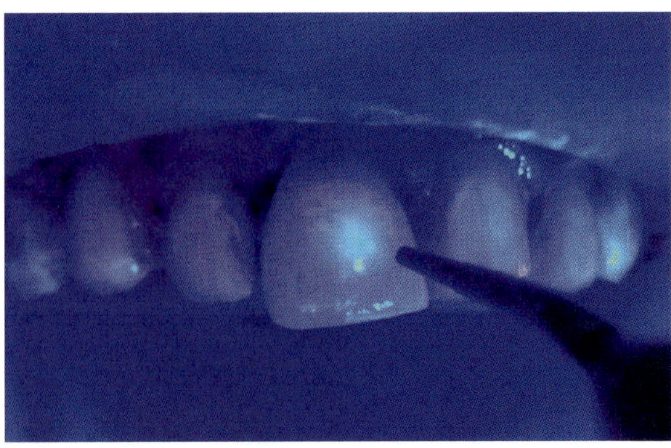

Fig. 4.48 After the position of the veneers is verified, the cement is cured using the "tack and wave" technique for 1–3 s

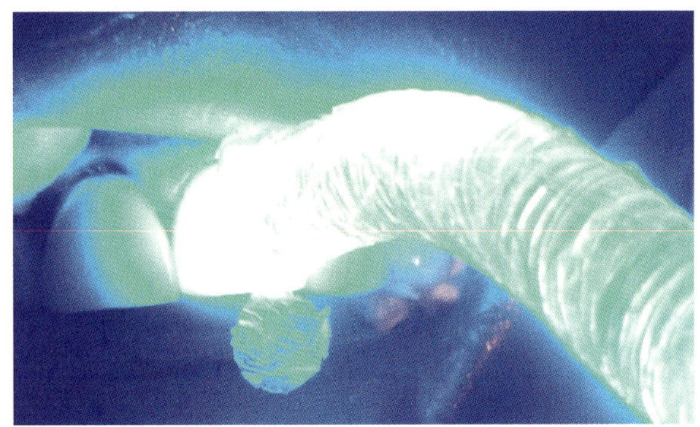

Fig. 4.49 The excess "tack-cured" cement being removed. The resin cement is only partially cured and is easy to remove in one clean piece. The hand instrument should be moved in an axial direction and not cervico-incisally to protect the fragile cement line

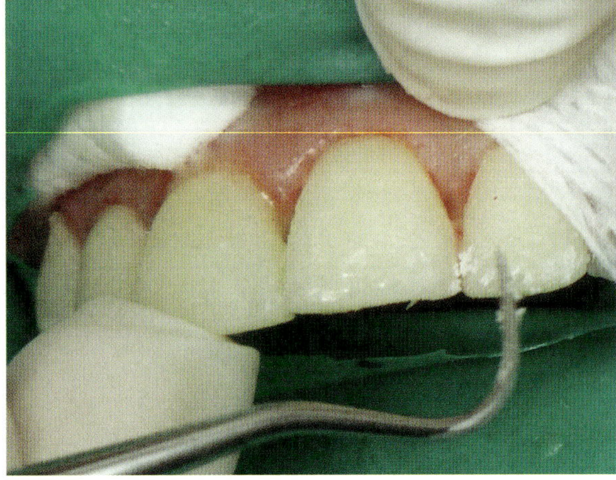

Fig. 4.50 Final curing of the cement

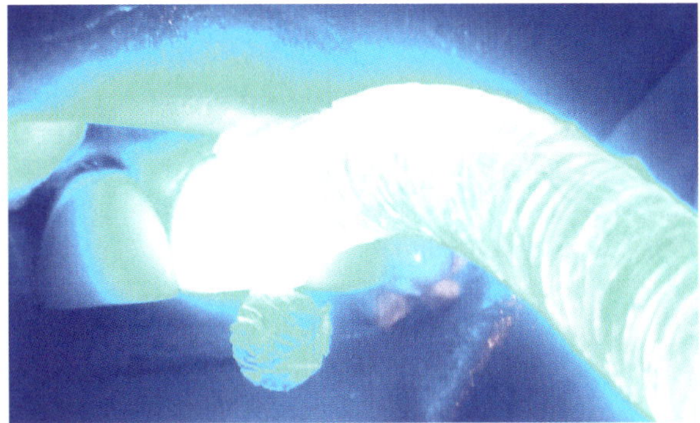

Fig. 4.51 A #12 scalpel blade is used to remove the remaining excess cement on the interproximal margins

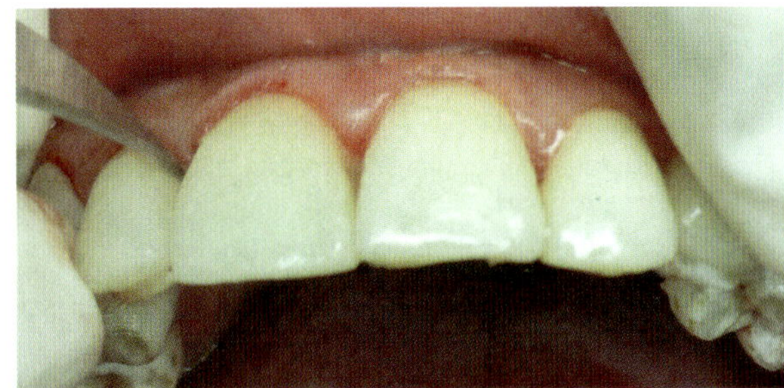

Fig. 4.52 The cemented veneers

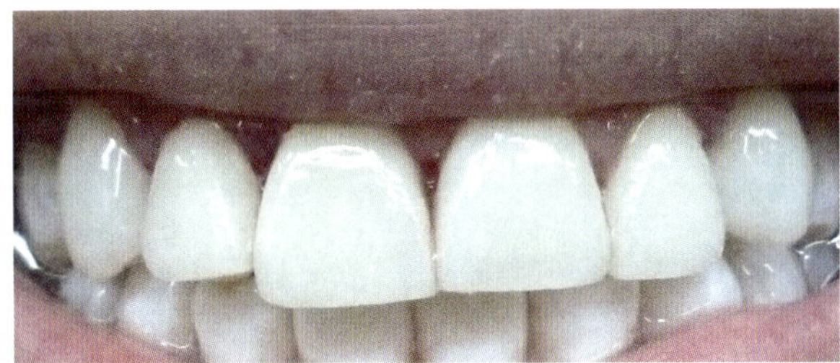

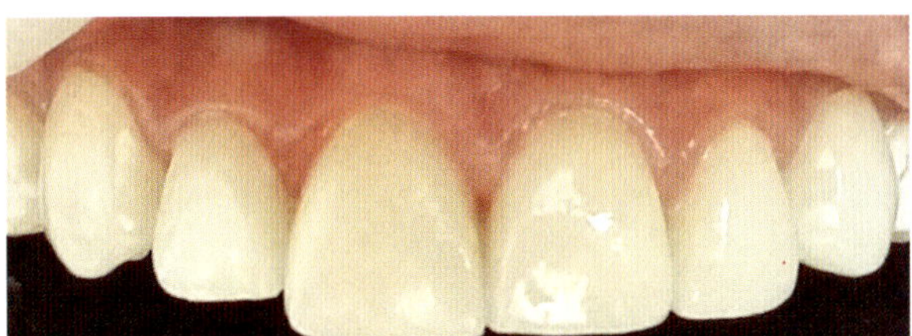

Fig. 4.53 At 3 weeks recall

4.4.3   Porcelain Crowns (Silica-Based Crowns)

4.4.3.1 Choosing the Right Cement

The recommended cements for porcelain crowns are the dual-cured resin cements to ensure complete polymerization underneath the thick ceramic even without the presence of light. The choice of resin cement will depend mainly on the degree of retention required. Some authors (Christensen 2007) recommend the use of self-etch resin cements and self-adhesive resin cements over total-etch resin cements as most crown preparations are in the dentin. Total-etch resin cements however can still be used for cementation of crowns as long as all precautions are taken to prevent overdrying and over-etching of the dentin which are the primary reasons for postoperative sensitivity.

Table 4.1 Recommendations for cementation of porcelain crowns

Clinical situation	Recommended cement
Crown preparations with minimal tooth retention (less than 4 mm height, crown preparations with more than 14° taper)	Self-etch resin cements (cements which are used in conjunction with self-etch primers (e.g., Panavia F 2.0, Bistite, ResiCem))
Crown preparations with adequate retention	Self-adhesive resin cement
Crowns that repeatedly come off	Self-etch resin cements

4.4.3.2 Clinical Case

Porcelain crowns (E-max) on teeth numbers 11, 21, and 22

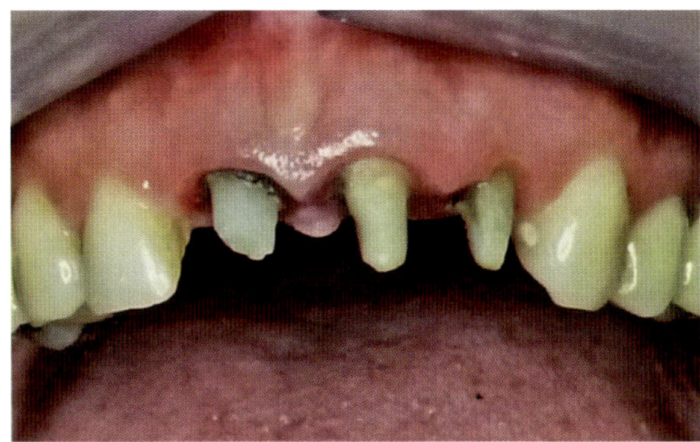

Fig. 4.54 Prepared teeth

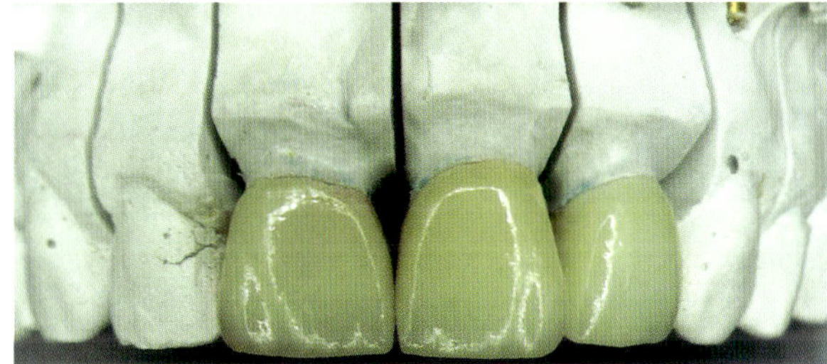

Fig. 4.55 The ceramic crowns on the working cast

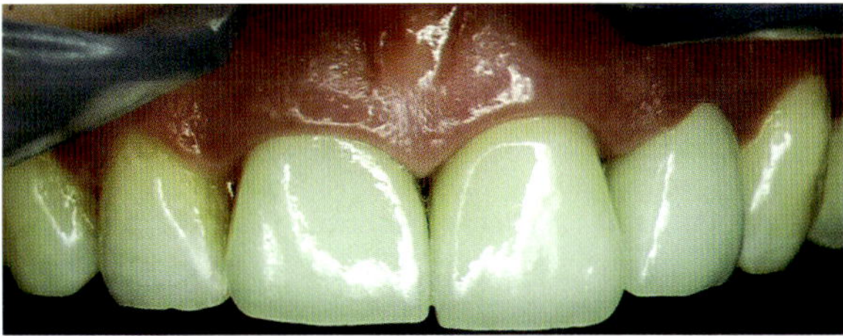

Fig. 4.56 Seating/trial fitting of the three crowns

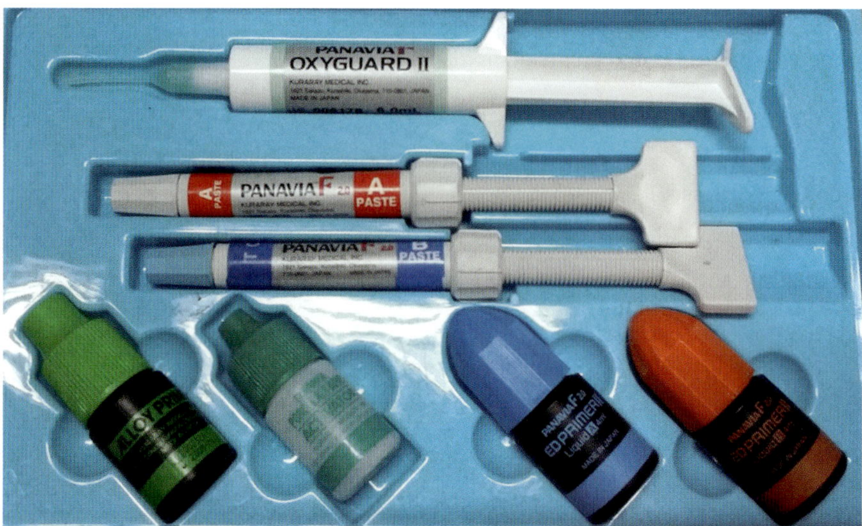

Fig. 4.57 Panavia F 2.0, a self-etch resin cement, is used to cement the crowns. Because of the small size of the prepared teeth, retention is compromised. Thus, a conventional self-etch resin cement is chosen over a self-adhesive resin cement

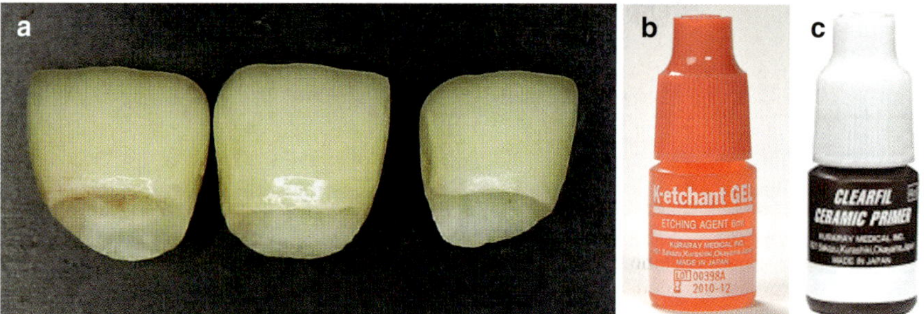

Fig. 4.58 Preparation of the restoration surface. (**a**) The internal surface of the crowns were sandblasted by the laboratory. (**b**) The internal surface was treated with K-etchant gel (phosphoric acid) for 5 s and then rinsed. (**c**) Clearfil ceramic primer (silanating agent) was applied on the internal surface of the crowns and lightly air-dried

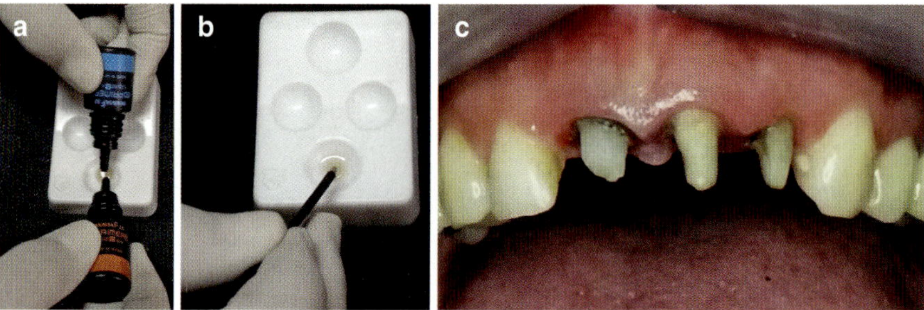

Fig. 4.59 Treatment of the tooth surface. (**a**) Equal amounts of ED Primer A and ED Primer B were dispensed in a mixing well (**b**) and were thoroughly mixed. (**c**) The primer was then applied on the prepared teeth and air-dried

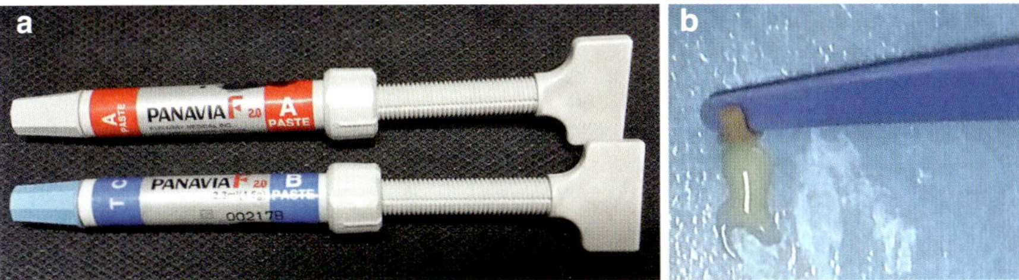

Fig. 4.60 Dispensing and mixing of the resin cement. (**a**) Panavia F 2.0 pastes A and B. (**b**) Equal amounts of pastes A and B were dispensed and thoroughly mixed using folding strokes to minimize air bubbles

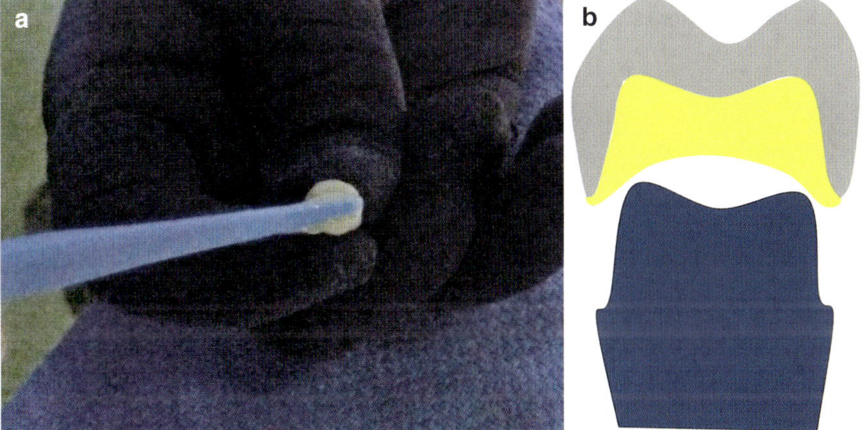

Fig. 4.61 (**a**) The resin cement is loaded into the crowns. The cement is agitated to remove air bubbles. (**b**) Diagram showing correct way of placing cement into the crown. It is not necessary to overfill the crown. The crown is filled with cement only halfway making sure that the margins are covered with cement

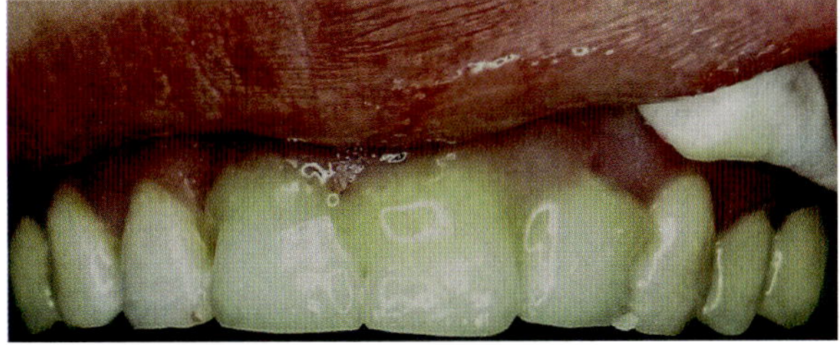

Fig. 4.62 The cements are seated slowly using light finger pressure. Strong abrupt loading force is avoided so as not to cause pressure from building up inside the crowns. This buildup might push the crown occlusally once seating pressure is removed resulting to improper seating of the crown and occlusal prematurities. The cement, especially on the margin areas, is tack cured for 1–2 s

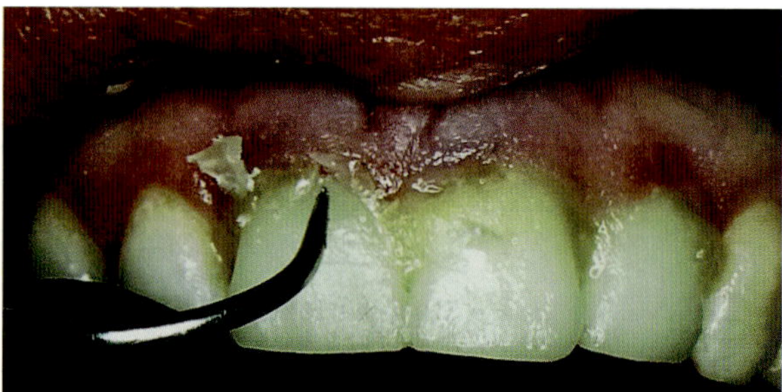

Fig. 4.63 The tack-cured excess cement is removed. The cement is then completely light cured for 20 s

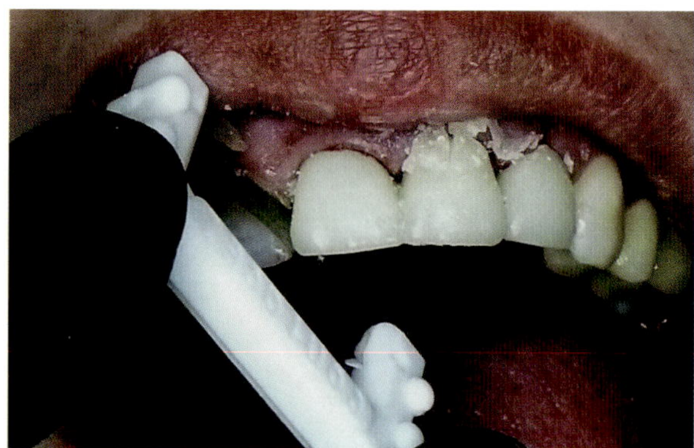

Fig. 4.64 A proximal adjuster (contact E-Z) is used to check and adjust the proximal fit of the crowns

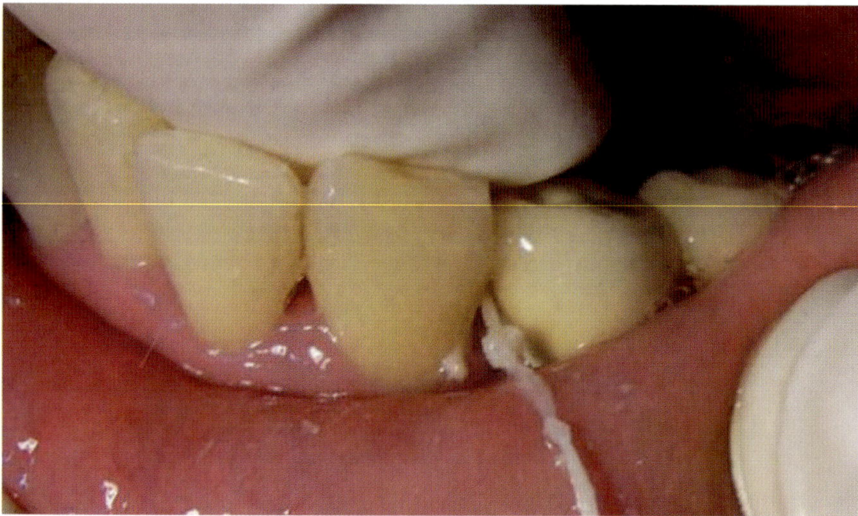

Fig. 4.65 A dental floss with a knot at the center is passed through the crowns to remove the remaining excess cement which might have been missed

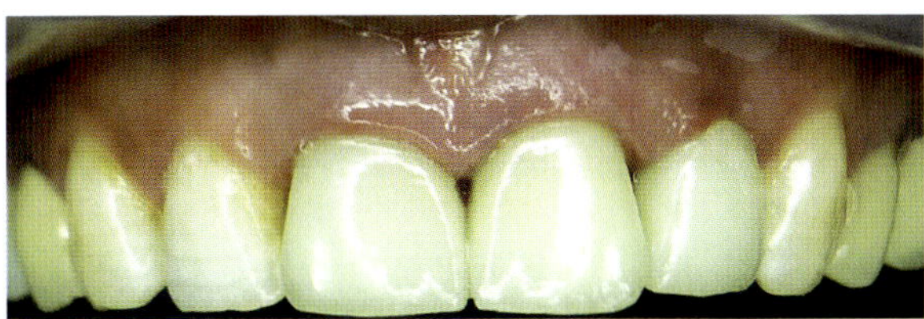

Fig. 4.66 The cemented crowns

4.4.3.3 Important Notes

1. Recommended cements for ceramic crowns are the dual-cured resin cements.
2. Dual-cured resin cements still require light polymerization to attain optimal curing properties.
3. The crown should be cemented using light, gradual pressure.
4. When loading the cement, the margins should be well coated with cement.
5. An oxygen barrier is sometimes used to protect the cement on the margins, while the self-curing polymerization is taking place.
6. Zirconia crowns and alumina-based crowns are NEVER etched with hydrofluoric acid nor silanated. For proper pretreatment of zirconia and alumina-based crowns, see Chap. 2.

4.4.4 Porcelain-Fused-to-Metal (PFM) Crowns

Resin cements are seldom used to cement PFM crowns. The usual cements for PFM are the glass-ionomer cements and even the zinc phosphate cements. Resin cements are only used for PFM crowns with compromised retention.

Cementation of porcelain-fused-to-metal crowns involves the same procedures as that of all-ceramic crowns except for the internal surface of the metal is treated with an alloy primer to enhance bonding with the resin cement.

Acknowledgments To our former students and now colleagues:
Drs. Louielyn Panganiban, Rosabelle Garcia, Isabella Limjap, and Mark Angelo Pablo for partly contributing to the text of this chapter.

References

Barceleiro MO, De Miranda MS, Dias KR, Sekito T Jr (2003) Shear bond strength of porcelain laminate veneer bonded with flowable composite. Oper Dent 28:423–428

Cagidiaco MC, Ferrari M et al (1996) Dentin contamination protection after mechanical preparation for veneering. Am J Dent 9:57–60

Chadwick RG, McCabe JF, Carrick TE (2008) Rheological properties of veneer trial pastes relevant to clinical success. Br Dent J 22:E11

Christensen GJ (2007) Should resin cements be used for every cementation? J Am Dent Assoc 138:817–819

Dietschi D (2002) Marginal and internal adaptation of Class II restorations after immediate or delayed composite placement. J Dent 30:259–269

Esmaili A, Saboury A, Ghassemi A (2007) The effect of flowable composite and resin cement on shear bond strength of porcelain veneer to enamel. J Islamic Den Assoc Iran 19:79–86

Geissberger MJ et al (2002) Simplified clinical procedure for fitting and removing inlays/onlays prior to cementation. J Prosthet Dent 87(4):395

Hornbrook D. Tack and wave technique: predictable veneer cementation. Surgical restorative resource from www.surgicalrestorative.com/articles/2012/tack-and-wave-technique. Accessed 18 June 2012

Magne Pascal KT (2005) Immediate dentin sealing improves bond strength of indirect restorations. J Prosthet Dent 94(6):511–519

McLaren EZ, Hamilton J (2007) Tips and tricks for the adhesive cementation of ceramic inlays, onlays and veneers. Inside Dentistry Volume 3 Issue 1. Available from www.dentalaegis.com/id/2007/01/lab-talk-tips-and-tricks-for-the-adhesive-cementation-of-ceramic-inlays-onlays-and-veneers. Accessed 15 December 2013

Munoz-Viveros C 20 Tips for resin veneer cements. J Cosmet Dentistry. From http://www.aacd.com/index.php?module=cms&page=773. Accessed 5 May 2012

Nikaido T, Takada T, Burrow MF, et al (1992) Early bond strengths of dual cured resin cements to enamel and dentin (in Japanese, English abstract) J. Jpn Dent Mater 11:910–915

Nikaido T, Nakaoki Y et al (2003) The resin coating technique. Effect of a single step bonding system on dentin bond strengths. J Adhes Dent 3:293–300

Pashley EL, Comer RW et al (1992) Dentin permeability: sealing the dentin in crown preparations. Oper Dent 17:13–20

Appendices

Glossary of Terms

Acidic monomer Active component of self-etch primers. These monomers simultaneously etch and prime the dentin and enamel, eliminating the need for a separate phosphoric acid etchant

Airborne particle abrasion Commonly known as *sandblasting*. The use of microfine aluminum oxide particles under air pressure (50–110 µm at 2.5 bar pressure) to render the ceramic surface rough and increase surface tension to enhance bonding to the resin cement

Alloy/metal primer Chemical solution that is painted on the internal surface of indirect restorations made of metal or with metal subsurface to increase the bond to resin cements prior to cementation

Conventional resin cements Resin cements that use a separate adhesive system, which requires multiple steps; pretreatment of both the involved tooth surfaces and internal surface of the restoration

Dentin primer Chemical solution consisting of a cofunctional monomer with both a hydrophobic end and hydrophilic end and a solvent/carrier, which can either be acetone, ethanol, or water. In simplified systems, the primer is either combined with an etchant to form the "self-etch" primer or combined with the adhesive to form the "self-priming" adhesive for total-etch or etch and rinse systems

Dual-cure polymerization Process of polymerization that occurs chemically through reaction with tertiary amine photoinitiators and through exposure to light

Feldspathic porcelain Low-strength silica-based porcelain, also known as veneering porcelain; the recommended ceramic for porcelain veneer restorations or as the veneering layer for high-strength core ceramics and porcelain-fused-to-metal restorations because of its high translucency and esthetic properties

Hybrid layer The layer formed by the intermingling of the primer and adhesive with the collagen fibrils of the dentin effectively sealing the opened dentinal tubules. The hybrid layer is the main mechanism of adhesion of resins to the dentin surface

© Springer-Verlag Berlin Heidelberg 2015
M. Sunico-Segarra, A. Segarra, *A Practical Clinical Guide to Resin Cements*,
DOI 10.1007/978-3-662-43842-8

Indirect or laboratory-fabricated composites Highly filled composite resins with microhybrid fillers and less organic matrix initially cured with light and secondarily cured either by heat or high-intensity light. Fabrication is entirely done by the laboratory

Inlay Is an intracoronal indirect restoration either made of metal, ceramic, or composite resin. Inlays are usually done when the decay or fracture is so extensive that the remaining tooth structure cannot adequately support the restoration, but does not involve any cusp, and a directly placed restoration such as amalgam or composite resin will compromise the structural integrity of the restored tooth

Interdental white tape Aka Teflon tape or plumber's tape. Commercially available thin white tape inserted between adjacent teeth to prevent them from bonding together during adhesive and cementation procedures

Leucite-reinforced porcelain Low- to moderate-strength silica-based porcelain commonly used as a veneering layer for high-strength core ceramics and porcelain-fused-to-metal restorations; flexural strength is somewhat higher than those of feldspathic porcelains as the leucite particles act to enhance resistance to crack propagation

Light-cure polymerization Polymerization process where the resin hardens through exposure to light usually in the wavelength of 400–480 nm, which is absorbed by the camphoroquinone initiator in the resin

Lithium disilicate porcelain Moderate-strength silica-based porcelain that can be used without a high-strength ceramic core or metal substructure. Indicated for onlays, inlays, and all-ceramic crowns and short-span bridges

MDP (10-methacryloyloxydecyl dihydrogen phosphate) Is a monomer which is a component of some self-etch adhesive systems and resin cements. It has been shown in several studies that MDP is the only monomer that can produce high bond strengths with zirconia- and alumina-based ceramic crowns. Sandblasting the internal surface of zirconia- and alumina-based crowns can increase further the bond strengths to resin cements

Onlay Is an indirect intracoronal restoration either made of metal, ceramic, or composite resin that involves one or more cusps of the tooth

Oxygen barrier A gel-like substance, usually glycerin based, that is applied on the surface of the setting dual-cured resin cement to prevent oxygen from interfering with polymerization

Phosphoric acid etchant Usually 36–37 % orthophosphoric acid. Used to create microporosities on enamel and demineralize the most superficial layer of dentin. The subsequently applied primer and bonding agent will fill up the microporosities created to form resin tags and the so-called hybrid layer in the dentin

Polymerization Chemical reaction by which monomers are converted to polymers resulting into a hardened resin paste

Porcelain etchant Is a chemical solution used to improve the adhesion between the ceramic restoration and the resin cement by creating microporosities on the ceramic, thereby increasing the surface energy for bonding. Most common porcelain etchant is *hydrofluoric acid* (in 2.5–10 % concentration). Etching of the internal surface of the ceramic restoration is usually done for 2–3 min followed by either ultrasonic cleaning for 5 min, steam cleaning, or cleaning with an alcohol solution to remove the white residue that forms after porcelain etching

Self-adhesive resin cements Resin cements that do not require pretreatment of the involved tooth surfaces. These cements contain acidic monomers and phosphate esters that render them self-adhesive

Self-cure polymerization Polymerization process where the resin polymerizes, sets, or hardens by purely chemical reaction. This process is initiated by tertiary amines present in the resin

Self-etch resin cements Conventional resin cements that require application of a self-etch primer on the involved tooth surface prior to cementation

Silane/silanating agent Is a coupling agent applied on the internal surface of ceramic and composite resin restorations to provide a more stable and durable bond with the resin cement

Tack and wave technique Cementation technique with resin cements where the restoration is seated on the tooth and cured for 1 s on the center with a small-diameter light guide followed by curing with a larger-diameter light guide waved about 1 inch from the restoration for about 3 min. The cement attains a semi-gel state, allowing the restoration to be initially seated without falling or drifting off, and it gives the cement a consistency that makes it easy to be removed or peeled off from the surface of the restoration

Total-etch resin cements Conventional resin cements that require phosphoric acid etching of the involved tooth surface and subsequent application of a self-priming adhesive prior to cementation. Also called etch-and-rinse cements

Tribochemical silicoating The process of coating the internal surface of the zirconia or alumina restoration with silica–aluminum by air abrading it with aluminum trioxide particles with silica to enhance bonding of zirconia or alumina ceramics to the resin cement

Zirconia crowns Crowns made of zirconium dioxide. Can either be a coping (to replace the metal substructure in porcelain-fused-to-metal crowns) or veneered with silica-based ceramics, such as feldspathic and leucite-reinforced ceramics, or can be monolithic zirconia, that is, the crown is made up entirely of zirconia. Zirconia crowns have very high compressive and tensile strengths. These crowns are not to be etched with hydrofluoric acid nor silanated

Examples of Resin Cements

Cement name	Mode of polymerization	Mechanism of adhesion	General indications (for more specific indications, please refer to Chaps. 3 and 4)	Manufacturer
Beauticem	Dual cure	Self-adhesive	Inlays, onlays, crowns and bridges, esthetic posts	Shofu
Biscem	Dual cure	Self-adhesive	Inlays, onlays, crowns and bridges, esthetic posts	Bisco
Bistite	Dual cure	Self-etch	Inlays, onlays, crowns and bridges, esthetic posts	Tokuyama
Breeze	Dual cure	Self-adhesive	Inlays, onlays, crowns and bridges, esthetic posts	Pentron
C&B Cement	Self-cure	Total-etch	Inlays, onlays, crowns and bridges, esthetic posts	Bisco
C&B Metabond	Self-cure	Total-etch	Inlays, onlays, crowns and bridges, esthetic posts	Parkell
Calibra	Dual cure	Total-etch	Inlays, onlays, crowns and bridges, esthetic posts	Dentsply
Calibra	Light cure (base paste only)	Total-etch	Veneers	Dentsply
Cement-It	Dual cure	Total-etch	Inlays, onlays, crowns and bridges, esthetic posts	Pentron
Choice 2	Light cure	Total-etch	Veneers	Bisco
Clear I Esthetic	Dual cure	Total-etch	Inlays, onlays, crowns and bridges	Kuraray
Clear I Esthetic Cement	Light cure	Total-etch	Veneers	Kuraray
Comspan	Self-cure	Total-etch	Inlays, onlays, crowns and bridges, esthetic posts	Dentsply
Dual Cement	Dual cure	Total-etch	Inlays, onlays, crowns and bridges, esthetic posts	Ivoclar
Duo Cement Plus	Dual cure	Total-etch	Inlays, onlays, crowns and bridges, esthetic posts	Coltene/ Whaledent
Duolink	Dual cure	Total-etch	Inlays, onlays, crowns and bridges, esthetic posts	Bisco
Duolink SE	Dual cure	Self-etch	Inlays, onlays, crowns and bridges, esthetic posts	Bisco
Embrace	Dual cure	Self-adhesive	Inlays, onlays, crowns and bridges, esthetic posts	Pulpdent

Cement name	Mode of polymerization	Mechanism of adhesion	General indications (for more specific indications, please refer to Chaps. 3 and 4)	Manufacturer
G-Cem	Dual cure	Self-adhesive	Inlays, onlays, crowns and bridges, esthetic posts	GC
ICem	Dual cure	Self-adhesive	Inlays, onlays, crowns and bridges, esthetic posts	Heraeus
Illusion	Dual cure	Total-etch	Inlays, onlays, crowns and bridges, esthetic posts	Bisco
Illusion	Light cure	Total-etch	Veneers	Bisco
Infinity	Dual cure	Total-etch	Inlays, onlays, crowns and bridges, esthetic posts	Den Mat
Maxcem	Dual cure	Self-adhesive	Inlays, onlays, crowns and bridges, esthetic posts	Kerr Sybron
Maxcem Elite	Dual cure	Self-adhesive	Inlays, onlays, crowns and bridges, esthetic posts	Kerr Sybron
Multilink	Dual cure	Self-adhesive	Inlays, onlays, crowns and bridges, esthetic posts	Ivoclar
Nexus 2	Dual cure	Total-etch	Inlays, onlays, crowns and bridges, esthetic posts	Kerr Sybron
Nexus 3	Dual cure	Total-etch	Inlays, onlays, crowns and bridges, esthetic posts	Kerr Sybron
NX 3	Light cure (single syringe)	Total-etch	Veneers	Kerr Sybron
Panavia F 2.0	Dual cure	Self-etch	Inlays, onlays, crowns and bridges, veneers, esthetic posts	Kuraray
ParaCem	Dual cure	Total-etch	Inlays, onlays, crowns and bridges, esthetic posts	Coltene/Whaledent
PermaFloDC	Dual cure	Total-etch	Inlays, onlays, crowns and bridges, esthetic posts	Ultradent
RelyX U200	Dual cure	Self-adhesive	Inlays, onlays, crowns and bridges, esthetic posts	3 M Espe
RelyX Veneer	Light cure	Total-etch	Veneers	3 M Espe
Resicem	Dual cure	Self-etch	Inlays, onlays, crowns and bridges, esthetic posts	Shofu
Resilute	Dual cure	Total-etch	Inlays, onlays, crowns and bridges, esthetic posts	Pulpdent

Cement name	Mode of polymerization	Mechanism of adhesion	General indications (for more specific indications, please refer to Chaps. 3 and 4)	Manufacturer
Smart Cem 2	Dual cure	Self-adhesive	Inlays, onlays, crowns and bridges, esthetic posts	Dentsply
Superbond	Self-cure	Total-etch	Inlays, onlays, crowns and bridges, esthetic posts	Sun Medical
Twinlock	Dual cure	Total-etch	Inlays, onlays, crowns and bridges, esthetic posts	Heraeus
Ultrabond Plus	Light cure	Total-etch	Veneers	Den Mat
Variolink 2	Dual cure	Total-etch	Inlays, onlays, crowns and bridges, esthetic posts	Ivoclar
Variolink Veneer	Light cure	Total-etch	Veneers	Ivoclar

Index

© Springer-Verlag Berlin Heidelberg 2015
M. Sunico-Segarra, A. Segarra, *A Practical Clinical Guide to Resin Cements*,
DOI 10.1007/978-3-662-43842-8

Printing: Ten Brink, Meppel, The Netherlands
Binding: Stürtz, Würzburg, Germany